LARGE PRINT

C -
6/3
W

Weil

Ask Dr. Weil

32740

PB

DATE DUE

Nov 8, 2003	
DISCARDED	

PRINTED IN U.S.A.

Also available
in Random House Large Print

EIGHT WEEKS TO OPTIMUM HEALTH

ASK DR. WEIL

Andrew Weil, M.D.

Edited by Steven Petrow

Published by Random House Large Print
in association with Ballantine Books
New York   1998

Copyright © 1997, 1998 by Great Bear Productions, LCC

All rights reserved under International and
Pan-American Copyright Conventions.
Published in the United States of America
by Random House Large Print
in association with Ballantine Books,
New York, and simultaneously in Canada
by Random House of Canada Limited, Toronto.
Distributed by Random House, Inc., New York.

This work was compiled from the "Ask Dr. Weil" Web site. It was previously published in 1997 by The Ballantine Publishing Group in six volumes entitled *Common Illnesses, Healthy Living, Natural Remedies, Vitamins and Minerals, Women's Health,* and *Your Top Health Concerns.*

---

*Library of Congress Cataloging-in-Publication Data
is available upon request.*

Random House Web Address: http://www.randomhouse.com/
Printed in the United States of America
FIRST LARGE PRINT EDITION

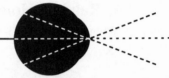

This Large Print Book carries the
Seal of Approval of N.A.V.H.

About "Ask Dr. Weil"

The "Ask Dr. Weil" program (www.drweil.com) features Andrew Weil, M.D., and is one of the top-rated health sites on the World Wide Web and is featured on Time Warner's Pathfinder Network. The recipient of many awards, the "Ask Dr. Weil" program features a daily Q&A with answers to a wide range of health questions, a daily poll, and the Doc Weil Database, which lets readers search hundreds of topics, including material from Dr. Weil's bestselling book *Natural Health, Natural Medicine.* The site also features a Referral Directory (practitioners from acupuncture to Trager work) and DocTalk, a live weekly chat with Dr. Weil. If you have additional questions for Dr. Weil, ask them on his Web site.

Acknowledgments

Richard Pine, Judith Curr, Elisa Wares, and Scott Fagan

Introduction

A little over two years ago I got on the information superhighway—as it was called then—with the launch of my interactive health program on the World Wide Web, "Ask Dr. Weil." The concept was both deceptively simple and revolutionary. From the outset, I took questions from readers like you and answered them daily on the Web. In the first week the program was "live"; we got about 1,000 questions. By last count we are getting about 60,000 questions a month from viewers like you.

That's the simple part!

At the end of each question, the program staff starts a discussion topic—known as a "message board" by my Internet readers—where you, other professionals, and I talk and argue about the issue of the day. Topics have ranged from the fairly sedate ("Best remedies for a cold?") to the hotly contested ("Is caffeine an addictive drug?"). What I like most about the message boards—and what I think you do, too—is the opportunity to break down the walls between physician and patient. And the information flow is not just one-way. I learn from you, too. Over the past two years, readers have made me aware of new remedies, therapies, and healthy foods.

I also host a live "call-in" program on "Ask Dr. Weil," where readers call me on an 800 number and ask their questions; all of this is then broadcast—live—on the Web around the globe. More than that, the Web site is a far-reaching yet close-knit community of people like you, who are taking an active role in staying healthy and who believe in my approach to health, wellness, and medicine. For me, this kind of real interactivity—not the bells and whistles kind you usually read about—is what makes "Ask Dr. Weil" so revolutionary.

Other parts of the site also draw in readers to learn and connect in new ways. Last year, concurrent with the publication of my book *Eight Weeks to Optimum Health,* we created the interactive, on-line version of the book, called "Eight Weeks to a Healthy America." Each week, I guide you through the program one step at a time, asking you to make a variety of changes in how you eat, how you exercise, what vitamins you take, and how you use your mind. You become a part of a community of real people who are doing it along with you. So far, tens of thousands of you have participated in "Eight Weeks to a Healthy America."

Many of you have also found great value in "The Vitamin Adviser." With all the supplements lining the store shelves, it's hard to know what vitamins and minerals you really need to take. Obviously, your needs depend on your age, your gender, your health history, and your lifestyle. "The Vitamin Adviser" designs a customized list of supplements just for you. You can build your profile and finally figure out how much of what you need and why. I think you'll find this a very useful "tool," as they say on the Web.

The book you're holding is a compilation of the Q&As that have appeared on the Web site. All of the questions contained in these pages came directly from readers. I think we've pretty much covered the health world from A to Z (or from abs to zinc). You'll find questions and answers here about natural remedies, common illnesses, women's health, diet and nutrition, mind-body science, and more.

You may have more questions. In that case, I urge you to visit us on-line at www.drweil.com. Once you're there it's easy to ask me a question. Basically you type it into a form, tell us who you are (or be anonymous) and . . . click. Your question is on its way to me.

Continued good luck and good health to you as you work toward optimum health in your life.

Andrew Weil, M.D.

Do I Need Abs of Steel?

Q:

It seems that I can't turn on the television anymore without seeing an infomercial for an abdominal exercising gizmo. Are any of these products really effective at helping a person "lose inches" and "shape the midsection"?

A:

Let me say at the start that washboard stomachs aren't necessarily desirable. Sure, they look good on slick magazine paper (and the TV screen), but they may not be healthy. A super-flat abdomen with tight, rippling muscles will restrict the motion of the intestines during digestion. It may also crimp the action of the diaphragm, which needs to move freely in order for you to breathe optimally. It's okay to be trim, but a well-toned abdomen should be yielding, not rigid.

The ab-gizmo makers are just the latest industry to capitalize on our society's obsession with lean bodies. In 1995, they sold $145 million worth of these devices.

Abdominal crunches in moderation can be helpful. They can strengthen the back as well as the abdominal muscles. They help reduce back pain by balancing and toning the muscles that support the spine. And they may help some people shape their midsections.

You don't need to buy an expensive apparatus to

work your abdominal muscles: a basic stomach crunch will do. Lie on the floor with knees bent, palms on your legs or on the floor, and feet comfortably apart. Keep your chin up (focus your eyes on the ceiling) and curl your body forward until your shoulders are a few inches off the floor. Hold, relax, and repeat. And remember to keep breathing.

It does make sense to pay attention to your body weight. If you are more than 20 percent heavier than your ideal weight, you may have increased risk of cardiovascular disease, diabetes, gallstones, some kinds of cancer, and osteoarthritis. Also note that body composition may be a more accurate way to determine your ideal weight than actuarial tables. Percentage of body fat is usually measured by weighing under water, but new computerized analysis is much simpler—and drier!

Remember: Spot reduction isn't the answer, whether you use those devices or not. The secret to losing weight won't cost you anything: eat less (especially less fat) and get more aerobic exercise. If you want to crunch your abs, that's okay, too.

Acupuncture for Fido or Felix?

Q:
Has acupuncture been used to treat cancer in dogs? If not for a cure, at least for pain reduction? Just curious. My beloved dog has inoperable cancer. There doesn't seem to be a lot of literature regarding this.

A:
Acupuncture has been used on animals, including dogs, for arthritis, dysplasia, degenerative nerve conditions, epilepsy, immune system suppression, gastrointestinal problems, and more. In fact, there's an increasing number of holistic veterinarians, and they use acupuncture a lot. This treatment has not been used for cancer in humans, though, and it's never been represented as a cancer treatment. It is, however, very helpful for pain reduction. I think turning to integrative medicine to help your companion is an excellent idea.

Acupuncture works on the principle that life-force energy, called chi (or qi), flows through the body along pathways (meridians) just below the skin's surface. These pathways connect the surface of the body with internal organs and regulate the flow of energy. Acupuncture uses tiny needles to stimulate or fatigue certain points along the meridians and relieve blockage, disperse pain, strengthen muscles and organs, and redirect energy flow.

There are also herbal and nutritional approaches that may help extend life and reduce symptoms in dogs with cancer. I used some of these for my Rhodesian Ridgeback, Coca, when she had bone cancer. I gave her extract of maitake and reishi mushrooms. Maitake, or *Grifola frondosa,* and reishi, *Ganoderma lucidum,* are potent immune boosters. You can find extracts of them in health food stores. I think they helped Coca live much longer and more comfortably than her conventional veterinarian had predicted. She did very well up until the end.

If you decide to see an acupuncturist for your pet, make sure that person has been trained in animal acupuncture. Animal anatomy is different from human.

You may also want to try some acupressure on your own. I'm sure a loving massage by you could do wonders to relieve your dog's pain. *Four Paws, Five Directions,* a book by veterinarian Cheryl Schwartz, offers a comprehensive approach to applying traditional Chinese medicine and acupressure techniques to animals. Try her step-by-step daily massage, which will stimulate your dog's meridians and relax you both.

Can Animal Hormones Harm Kids?

Q:
A friend told me her nine-year-old daughter already has had her first period, as have most of her classmates! She says it's because of the estrogen they consume from additives in dairy and beef. Is this true? Are these girls typical?

A:
You're correct that the onset of menstruation has been getting progressively earlier among girls in the United States. No one is sure why, but one possibility is that commercially produced meat and milk products contain residues of growth-promoting hormones. These have estrogenic activity, so they could stimulate early menstruation.

Some years ago, there was an epidemic of premature puberty in very young girls (under four years old) in Puerto Rico. This was traced to consumption of chicken carrying unusually high residues of estrogenic hormones.

Another disturbing possibility is that many environmental pollutants, including some pesticides and plastics, may act like estrogens in the body. Eating soy foods may offer protection from them.

There's reason to be concerned about early onset of menstruation, because it's a factor of significant risk for breast cancer. Women who menstruate early will have more years of exposure to their own estrogens, which stimulate the cells of the breasts and reproductive system to proliferate.

I would minimize the amount of animal food fed to children, or use only organically produced meat, poultry, or dairy products certified to be free of hormones. And try to get the kids to eat tofu!

What's in Your Antioxidant Cocktail?

Q:
What vitamins should I be taking on a regular basis?

A:
I get asked about the antioxidant "cocktail" perhaps more than about any other subject. You can really help your body by taking protective antioxidants, nutrients that protect tissues by blocking the chemical reactions by which many toxins cause harm. One way to go about it is to increase your consumption of fresh fruits and vegetables. You can also take supplements.

Here is the formula I use myself and recommend to my patients:

- *Vitamin C:* 1,000 to 2,000 milligrams two to three times a day. Your body can absorb this vitamin more easily in a soluble powder form than in a large tablet. I take a dose of vitamin C with breakfast and dinner, and, if I can remember, another before bed. Plain ascorbic acid may irritate a sensitive stomach, so take it with food or look for a buffered or nonacidic form.
- *Vitamin E:* 400 to 800 IU a day. People under forty should take 400 IU a day; people over forty, 800 IU. Since vitamin E is fat soluble, it must be taken with food to be absorbed. Also, natural vitamin E (d-alpha-tocopherol) is much better than

the synthetic form (dl-alpha-tocopherol). I usually take vitamin E at lunch. Make sure the product contains the other tocopherols, especially gamma, which offers protection that alpha-tocopherol does not.

- *Selenium:* 200 to 300 micrograms a day. Selenium is a trace mineral with antioxidant and anticancer properties. Selenium and vitamin E facilitate each other's absorption, so take them together. Vitamin C may interfere with the absorption of some forms of selenium, so take them separately. Doses above 400 micrograms a day may not be healthy.
- *Mixed carotenes:* 25,000 IU a day. I take mixed carotenes as a supplement with my breakfast. I recommend a natural form—easily found in health food stores. Men: read the label to make sure it gives you lycopene, the red pigment in tomatoes that helps prevent prostate cancer.

All in all, this is a simple formula that will not cost you too much trouble or money.

Is Aspartame Dangerous?

Q:
I think I've had an adverse reaction to aspartame. I've used NutraSweet for fifteen years, usually consuming six to eight packets a day. Now I have reduced motor control of my arms and hands. Is there a link? What do you recommend?

A:
First of all, I would stop using NutraSweet. Although the manufacturer portrays aspartame as a gift from nature, and its two components do occur naturally, aspartame itself does not. Like all artificial sweeteners, aspartame has a peculiar taste. Because I have seen a number of patients—mostly women—who report headaches from using it, I don't view it as biologically inert. Some women also find that aspartame aggravates PMS. There are no proven long-term toxic effects, but there is a lot of suspicion.

In general, I think you're better off using moderate amounts of sugar. People who use NutraSweet to control their weight should know there's not a shred of evidence that the availability or use of artificial sweeteners has helped anyone to lose weight. Think about it: You have pie à la mode for dessert (about 495 calories), and then use a packet of NutraSweet for your coffee (saving 18 calories). There's something wrong with that calculation. Also, remember that aspartame turns up in unexpected items. Recently, on an airplane, I was given some mints that were sweetened with aspartame. Most people wouldn't have noticed it in the fine print on the label.

As for your motor troubles, I would advise going to a neurologist for an evaluation. Your condition may be unrelated to aspartame, although there is some anecdotal evidence indicating a link.

Treatment for Athlete's Foot?

Q:
My feet are itchy. Is grapefruit seed extract really as good for athlete's foot as the guy at the health food store claims?

A:
Athlete's foot is a fungal infection of the skin, related to jock itch and ringworm. As you probably know, it thrives in moist, warm, dark places, so one of the best treatments I can recommend is exposing your feet to fresh air and sunlight. Keep them clean and dry—and wear sandals if you can.

I've also heard a lot of positive testimonials about grapefruit seed extract, which is available at health food stores. It is reported to have significant antifungal effects. Apply the extract (full strength) two to three times a day to the affected area.

Tea tree oil, extracted from the leaves of *Melaleuca alternifolia,* a tree native to Australia, is another home remedy that works as well as or better than over-the-counter medications like Tinactin and Lotrimin. Apply a light coating of this product to the affected area three or four times a day, and continue to apply it for two weeks after the infection seems to have disappeared. You want to make sure the fungus is eradicated. Tea tree oil will also clear up fungal infections of the toenails or fingernails, conditions that are usually difficult to cure, even with strong systemic antibiotics. It's also effective for ringworm and jock itch as well as bacterial infections of the skin. You'll find tea tree oil products at health food and herb stores. Be sure to select ones that are 100 percent tea tree oil.

Do B-12 Boosters Work?

Q:
What do you think of taking B-12 to boost energy? Some friends of mine get shots regularly and say the vitamin works wonders.

A:
B-12 works in the body by helping the bone marrow regenerate red blood cells. The vitamin has been linked to protection against heart disease, and against mental deterioration such as memory loss. People use it to boost their energy, to recuperate from frequent partying with alcohol, and to revitalize themselves during menstruation.

Many people take vitamin B-12 shots as a quick way to pump up their energy level. I see this particularly among entertainers and theater people before performances. But most of them aren't deficient in B-12, so the shots are acting as very effective placebos. A placebo is a medicine or drug that doesn't have any direct therapeutic effect, but because of belief in its effectiveness, the patient experiences benefit. Placebo responses can be extremely powerful, and B-12 shots can definitely elicit them.

Most people I know who get B-12 shots say the first one filled them with a warm glow and a flush of energy. They felt terrific. But subsequent injections don't usually measure up. That's typical of placebos. Extreme fatigue can be a symptom of B-12 deficiency, but that needs to be confirmed by blood tests.

People take B-12 in the form of shots because it's not always easily absorbed through the stomach, and it needs to be combined with calcium to be useful to the body. So injections are the most effective way to get it into your system. If you hate shots, you can take the vitamin as a nasal spray, a nasal gel, or a lozenge you put under your tongue. You can also get it in a time-release formula combined with sorbitol for better absorption through the small intestine.

It's not hard to get enough B-12 in an ordinary diet. The body gets this vitamin almost exclusively from animal sources, such as liver, pork, milk, and eggs. Vegetarians, particularly vegans, are at risk for deficiency, especially vegan children. Many older people have trouble absorbing the vitamin from foods. B-12 deficiency results in pernicious anemia, which can produce such symptoms as weakness, apathy, light-headedness, shortness of breath, numbness in the extremities, and loss of balance. There may also be accompanying psychiatric changes such as paranoia and depression. In the elderly, B-12 deficiency can cause memory loss and disorientation that may look like Alzheimer's disease. All these symptoms can usually be reversed with supplemental B-12.

Experiment as you wish. B-12 is effective in very small doses, but has been found to be harmless even in amounts much higher than the 6 micrograms recommended daily.

Plagued by an Aching Back?

Q:
What do I do for lower back pain?

A:
Chronic back pain is often caused by unbalanced nervous control of the musculature, which triggers muscle contraction, reduction of normal blood supply, and inflammation. In most cases, it's not directly caused by structural injury, although injury can create a focal point for the effects of neuromuscular imbalance.

What you're feeling is the end result of a chain of nervous system events that starts in your brain and leads to pain in your back. Because the nervous system is connected to the mind and the emotions, healing is best directed there, often the root of the trouble. This isn't to say that your pain is all in your head, but rather that the vicious cycle of muscle spasm may have an emotional root. John Sarno, M.D., calls most cases of chronic back pain "tension myositis syndrome," referring to psychosomatic inflammation of the muscles. He has a great book on the subject called *Healing Back Pain*.

So rather than looking to chiropractors, osteopaths, acupuncturists, or massage practitioners to cure the pain, I'd try to understand the real nature of the problem and consider mental and emotional changes. Sometimes it may do the trick just to understand that the pain can depart once your brain stops sending the wrong messages to your back. Think about restructuring the patterns of thinking, feeling, and managing stress that lead your nervous system to spasm.

You can take steps to strengthen your back and improve the health of the muscles that contribute to the pain. Yoga is a wonderful way to improve flexibility and balance your nervous system. Stretches that target your hamstrings are a good way to make sure your back gets the support it needs. Abdominal strengthening exercises will also help.

The way you sit is important, too, especially if you spend long days at a computer or a desk. Sit a bit forward on your chair, with your knees comfortably apart and heels on the floor, your pelvis rotated slightly forward with your body balanced on top. If you place a rolled-up towel under your tailbone, it will help you achieve a good sitting posture. Don't puff out your chest; that's hard on your back, too.

There may also be a link between back pain and diet. One study found that arteries narrowed by atherosclerosis—avoidable with a low-fat diet—can't deliver as much blood to the lower back, and this affects disks, muscles, and nerves.

If you have an episode of acute lower back pain, use ice on the area as soon as you can. Chiropractic manipulation has also been shown to help. And keep in mind that almost everyone who suffers from acute back pain recovers in about a month with or without treatment.

How Safe Are Barbecues?

Q:
Our family is planning a couple of BBQs. Are there dangers to grilling?

A:
We know that charcoal grilling produces carcinogenic smoke from the high-temperature cooking of foods containing fat and protein (hot dogs, hamburgers, and chicken, to name some of your likely favorites) and unhealthy chemical changes in the outer layers of flesh foods. My two top recommendations: Don't inhale, and get used to cutting off any black or charred parts. Also, new research indicates that marinating meats for four hours greatly reduces their carcinogenicity on the grill.

Never use charcoal-lighting fluid or those self-lighting packages of charcoal; they both put residues from toxic chemicals into the food. I always use a "chimney lighter," in which a small amount of newspaper is ignited to get the coals burning.

I've noticed the trend toward more gourmet barbecuing—specifically, with mesquite briquettes. They're no better or worse than conventional briquettes, and the market for them is decimating the mesquite forests of the Southwest. On the other hand, I read recently that more people than ever before are using gas grills. That's good news for the environment.

By the way, fish or vegetables are great when grilled. Here's a recipe I often use:

Grilled Vegetables

Make a marinade of equal parts sake (or dry vermouth), olive oil, and Japanese soy sauce (shoyu). Add a few mashed garlic cloves and some hot pepper sauce if desired. Cut vegetables (onions, carrots, mushrooms, zucchini, red and green peppers, eggplants) into bite-size pieces and toss in the marinade to coat well. Let sit for thirty minutes while the grill is heating. Drain veggies and thread on skewers in artful order, then grill till they become tender and begin to brown. Serve with rice.

Better Treatments for Bee Stings?

Q:
A bumblebee and I got into a little rumble the other day and I ended up with a stinger in my lower leg. Never did find the stinger, but the area around the sting has gotten quite red and infected. My doc has put me on an antibiotic (cephalexin, 500 milligrams twice a day) for five days. Since I try to use antibiotics only as a last resort, what are the other options for insect stings?

A:
You're wise to avoid overdoing the antibiotics. If your body can beat an infection on its own, it will be more competent to combat future threats. If you override the system with an antibiotic right away, you weaken your own immunity. (There's also the danger of antibiotic resistance. Over time, frequent use of antibiotics leads to the breeding of more virulent bacteria that aren't fazed by existing treatments.)

What to do? Start by using hot compresses on the sting area. The heat dilates the blood vessels and increases healing blood flow to the site of the infection. Also, treat the inflammation locally with full-strength tea tree oil, which is a very effective topical antiseptic. (The oil is extracted from the leaves of *Melaleuca alternifolia,* a tree native to Australia.) Third, do a course of echinacea. Echinacea (*Echinacea purpurea* and related species), familiar to gardeners as purple coneflower, is a natural antibiotic and immune-system enhancer. Try a dropperful of tincture of echinacea in water four times a day for ten days or so. Take at least 1,000 milligrams of vitamin C twice a day, too.

Only if the infection continues to spread would I then use strong antibiotics. The cephalexin your doctor prescribed would be one choice. It's a semi-synthetic antibacterial, similar to penicillin, originally derived from a microorganism. This is a big gun, so wait a bit and try the other measures first.

As for treatment, for decades the advice concerning the proper way to remove the bee's stinger was to scrape it out with something like a blunt knife or a credit card. According to a recent study, you should grab the stinger and yank it out as fast as you can. Why the change? According to researchers at the University of California in Riverside, if you pluck out the stinger before all the venom is pumped out of it, you'll wind up with a smaller, less painful welt. But you have to act instantaneously to make a difference. The only problem is that while honeybees always leave a stinger, bumblebees rarely do. That's probably why you couldn't find it. To ease the pain and inflammation, ice the area immediately and then apply a paste made with baking soda and water.

Betting or Bailing on Beta-Carotene?

Q:
I've started to take 20,000 IU of beta-carotene a day per your suggestion. Recently I have read that beta-carotene supplements, even in these modest quantities, can be toxic. What is your latest opinion on the subject?

A:
Beta-carotene is not toxic, and there are no studies that suggest it may be. We do have some new information on the supplement, however, that shows it's not the panacea some people had hoped.

The interest in beta-carotene went mainstream after about two dozen studies showed that people with lots of beta-carotene-rich fruits and vegetables in their diets got less cancer and heart disease. As one of the vitamins that neutralize "free radical" molecules in the body, beta-carotene seemed to make sense as a preventive to oxidative damage leading to cancer.

But the results of giving the vitamin as a supplement were not all encouraging. A Finnish study reported 18 percent more cases of lung cancer among heavy smokers who took beta-carotene supplements. Then National Cancer Institute researchers halted a study on the effects of beta-carotene and vitamin A. Smokers taking the supplements had 28 percent more instances of lung cancer than those taking the placebo.

And a twelve-year study of 22,000 physicians found no evidence that beta-carotene supplements were protective against cancer and heart disease.

It's important to note that none of these studies showed that beta-carotene caused cancer. They weren't designed to ask that question. But they do indicate that beta-carotene fails to prevent cancer among smokers. No one is certain why. Some researchers point out that antioxidants can promote free radicals under certain circumstances rather than keeping them under control—and perhaps smoking triggers this action.

It's likely that cancer was already established in the people who were diagnosed with it during these trials. No one believes that antioxidants can cure existing cancers. But study after study has shown the protective effect of high levels of beta-carotene in the blood—and of large amounts of fruits and vegetables in the diet. It is probably not beta-carotene alone that is responsible. It could be the whole family of carotenoid pigments. (And so far, we don't have findings on the effects of beta-carotene in women. The Women's Antioxidant and Cardiovascular Study is continuing despite the negative findings in men.)

We know of about five hundred carotenoids, the family of substances that the body converts into vitamin A. I recommend taking advantage of them all. Eat a diet rich in fruits and vegetables, especially peaches, melons, mangoes, sweet potatoes, squash, pumpkins, tomatoes, and dark leafy greens. And if you cannot include enough of these in your diet, you may want to take a supplement. I recommend a *mixed carotene* supplement, such as Rainbow Light's Food 4 Life or Schiff's Beta Complete, which contain lycopene, lutein, alpha-carotene, and zeaxanthin, as well as beta-carotene. Take one capsule a day. Men: read labels to be sure the products contain lycopene, the red pigment in tomatoes; recent research shows it can help prevent prostate cancer.

Natural Methods of Birth Control?

Q:

I have been on the Pill for eight years. I'm tired of the mood swings, the increase in yeast infections, etc. A close friend uses a natural method that involves the monitoring of vaginal discharge together with an awareness of stages of her cycle, and she manages to avoid having intercourse during ovulation time. I have decided—with my husband's agreement—to try this. Do you know anything about this natural method?

A:

I think it's a good idea to go off the Pill if you can find other ways to practice contraception. The current generation of oral contraceptives are safer than those of the past, because they use lower doses of hormones. But you are still exposing the body to the very general effects of hormones, rather than getting just the specific effect on fertility that you desire. High levels of female sex hormones favor the development of cancer of the breast and of the reproductive system. And while there aren't any data clearly linking oral contraceptives to a higher risk of cancer, there is reason for caution.

Oral contraceptives also increase the risk of blood clots, and many women experience side effects such as nausea, breast tenderness, fluid retention, weight gain, and depression. The Pill reduces interest in sex over time, although triphasic versions, which vary the amount of synthetic progesterone and estrogen over the month, have less of this effect. If you smoke, have a family history of breast cancer, have a history of benign breast disease, did not have a first child until after age thirty-five, are over forty-five and still menstruating, or are at increased risk of cervical cancer because of multiple sex partners, I'd definitely say stay off the Pill.

If a woman becomes very aware of her body's cycles and pays attention to things like her temperature and the texture of her cervical mucus, I think it's possible for her to rely on a natural method. Certainly there are advantages, because a lot of women can't tolerate the side effects of the Pill.

You do need to recognize, however, that the natural method is less reliable and requires conscientious effort by both partners. The calendar rhythm method is least reliable. Measuring the woman's basal body temperature each morning is more accurate, as is watching for changes in the texture and amount of cervical mucus. A combination of these techniques is the most effective, but even with training in ways to monitor ovulation, the failure rate is still about 10 percent a year. Tracking ovulation is easier for some women than others, depending on the nature of their cycle.

But the natural method isn't the only way to go if you decide not to take the Pill. You can also choose condoms, foam and condoms, a contraceptive sponge, a diaphragm, or a cervical cap, which is similar to a diaphragm but can be left in the vagina longer.

Black-Eye Blues?

Q:
About three days ago I received a black eye while playing football. The swelling is down, but what is the best thing I can do to get the discoloration out of my eye? Is there any type of lotion that will speed up the healing process and remove the black and purple ring?

A:
A black eye is just a big bruise that happens to be in a very noticeable place. The first thing to do—which it sounds as if you've already done—is put cold on it. Immediately. That keeps the swelling down and may reduce the amount of bruising.

It is possible to speed up the healing process by taking the pineapple enzyme bromelain. You can buy bromelain in capsule form in health food stores. It is absorbed through the digestive tract and promotes healing of tissue injuries. Take 200 to 400 milligrams three times a day on an empty stomach (not within two hours of eating). A few individuals have allergic reactions to bromelain; discontinue if you get any itching.

Homeopathic arnica would also probably be a good idea, because it helps the body recover faster from trauma. Buy *Arnica montana* in 30x potency at a health food store, and let the tablets dissolve under your tongue. (Do not handle them. Shake them into the bottle cap and then toss them in your mouth.) Take four tablets immediately, then four every hour while awake the first day. The second day, cut back to four tablets every two hours; then four tablets four times a day. Continue the treatment four to five days. You may also want to rub some arnica tincture on the bruise, making sure to keep the arnica out of the eye itself.

In the meantime, keep smiling, and come up with a really enthralling story about your football adventure. You might also wear sunglasses!

Blood in My Stool?

Q:
*My boyfriend has just told me that he noticed blood in
his stool and in the toilet after having a bowel movement. He is afraid to call the doctor and insists he'll
wait and see if it happens again. I'm worried, though.
What could this be symptomatic of?*

A:
You're wise to pay attention. But your boyfriend may
be right about waiting until it happens again. If he's in
his twenties or thirties, the cause could be a number
of things—none of them likely to be terribly serious.
Hemorrhoids and ulcers can put blood in your stool.
An inflammatory condition called diverticulitis in the
colon could also be the cause.

In younger people, the most common reason for
blood in the stool is a hemorrhoid or fissure very near
the anus. There is also the possibility—if there is also
pain—that the cause is inflamed rectal tissue from a
sexually transmitted disease such as gonorrhea or
herpes. In general, bright red blood is coming from
a site close to the anus. Blood from higher up in the
digestive tract, such as from a bleeding ulcer, will
look black and tarry. Small amounts of blood leaking
into the gastrointestinal tract can be invisible or "occult." Doctors use a simple color test to reveal occult
blood in a tiny amount of stool obtained from a rectal

examination, and this should be done as part of every physical exam.

Older people should be very alert to blood in the stool because it can be a sign of colon cancer and always should be investigated. Colon cancer is curable only in its early stages, so it's very important to catch it right away. In this case it would be prudent to have a sigmoidoscopy. A sigmoidoscope is a long tube with a light at the end, which allows your doctor to get a direct look at the lining of the colon just above the anus, where most cancers arise. It can reveal polyps—mushroom-shaped growths that can be precancerous—as well as early malignant growths. There's also colonoscopy, a similar but more elaborate procedure to examine the entire colon with a fiberoptic scope. Other signs of colon cancer that might accompany blood in the stool are changes in bowel habits and in shape or consistency of stools.

Does Blue-Green Algae Boost Energy?

Q:

I'm curious about the blue-green algae thing. I was a total disbeliever in the high energy and healing claims many people reported to me, but I was worn down by friends and started taking it. It worked! What do you know and think about this?

A:

Frankly, I don't have any firsthand experience with blue-green algae. Like you, I've heard testimonials from people about its energy-boosting effects. According to what I've read, there is very little research on the chemistry or pharmacology of blue-green algae, but I found one unsettling paper indicating that the species used for commercial purposes is capable of producing liver and nerve toxins, which could be unhealthy in long-term use. Many users report drug-like stimulation from these products. Until I know what's responsible for that effect, I'm not going to recommend them. I've seen dozens of sites on the Web and many print advertisements promoting blue-green algae as a wonder food and an incredible business opportunity. Caveat emptor. I'd say wait and see on this. If it works for you, use it, but keep your eye out for new information.

If low energy is a problem for you, you could consider using ginseng, a natural tonic. Used on a regular basis, ginseng increases energy, vitality, sexual vigor, and provides resistance to all kinds of stress. It is non-toxic but Asian ginseng (*Panax ginseng*) can raise blood pressure and is more of a stimulant. I often recommend American ginseng (*Panax quinquefolius*) to people who are chronically ill and to those lacking in vitality.

Beating the Bottle Naturally?

Q:
What natural herbs have proven effective in battling alcoholism or helpful in curbing the craving for alcohol?

A:
Alcohol can produce true addiction, marked by intense craving, tolerance, and withdrawal. It's a powerful drug, and dependence on it is very resistant to treatment.

A couple of years ago, there was a flurry of excitement over reports that kudzu (*Pueraria*) from the south of China was effective as a treatment for alcohol dependence. It's sometimes used as a traditional remedy, and a preparation of the plant was found to reduce cravings for alcohol in strains of hamsters that were bred to be alcoholic. You can find a medicinal preparation of kudzu in Chinese herb stores.

Other than kudzu, I really don't know of any herbal methods for dealing with alcoholism. I'd start by making sure you have good nutrition. In particular, take B vitamins to make up for the B-vitamin deficiency alcoholism can cause. I would suggest one B-100 B-complex a day. Learn other methods of relaxation—like yoga or meditation—to replace alcohol. And get out there and exercise. I would also take two capsules of milk thistle (*Silybum marianum*) twice a day. It protects the liver.

I think the best bet for treating alcoholism is to go to an addiction treatment program. It's really difficult to deal with alcoholism without outside help. For one thing, there's tremendous social pressure to drink— and to drink too much. Consider going to a counseling center or Alcoholics Anonymous, or entering a residential program.

Lower Your Risk for Breast Cancer?

Q:

What specific things can women do to reduce the risk of breast cancer? It's well publicized that early breast-feeding is helpful. Can you give specific dietary recommendations or other suggestions? Thanks.

A:

Breast cancer results from a complex interaction of genetic and environmental factors. While we do not know all the details of its origin, we can make specific recommendations for lifestyle changes that will reduce risk. Some of these are intended to reduce estrogen production in the body or limit exposure to foreign estrogens. Those hormones stimulate breast cells to grow and divide, increasing the chance of malignant transformation. Other recommendations are aimed at strengthening the body's defenses.

Women who begin menstruating early have a higher risk of breast cancer, as do those who reach menopause late. Such women are exposed to estrogen for longer periods of time. Having a first baby at a younger age and breast-feeding both lessen the risk of breast cancer, probably by interrupting the menstrual cycle and reducing lifetime estrogen exposure. You may not be able to change much here, but you can make choices about your diet that will affect the amount of estrogen in your body.

Animal fats contribute to increased estrogen levels in the body, and a low-fat diet has been shown to help guard against breast cancer. Commercially raised animal foods often contain residues of estrogenic hormones given to animals as growth promoters. If you are a carnivore, you should check out Laura's Lean Beef at (800) ITS LEAN (487-5326). Laura Freeman runs a family farm outside Winchester, Kentucky, and all the beef is hormone- and antibiotic-free.

Soy products such as tofu, tempeh, and miso, which are full of weak, plant-based estrogens, lower cancer risk, perhaps because they occupy estrogen receptors, protecting them from stronger forms of the hormone (including many environmental pollutants). Compounds in cabbage block stronger surges of estrogen from other sources. Compounds in broccoli, kale, and collard greens also may be helpful.

On the other hand, alcohol, even in moderate usage, can increase estrogen production in susceptible women.

Regular, moderate exercise—four hours a week—reduced breast cancer risk before menopause by an average of 58 percent in one study. Researchers believe it lowers estrogen production. After menopause, exercise may still help by lessening body fat, another factor in estrogen exposure.

So the most important thing to think about is protecting the overall health and well-being of your body. Exercise regularly. Minimize your exposure to environmental estrogenic pollutants by eating low on the food chain. Especially limit your intake of commercially raised meats, dairy products, and eggs. Eat lots of organic fruits, vegetables, and soy foods and plenty of fiber to keep estrogen levels under control and protect your genes from damage. Also, take antioxidants to guard against deleterious mutations and protect immune defenses.

If you know you're at high risk, take two tablespoons of ground flaxseed on your cereal or in your juice every day. Flaxseed reduces the rate of growth of tumors in rats and lowers the chance of cancer's getting started in the first place.

Finally, note that the role of psychological factors in breast cancer is not at all clear. Grief and depression may suppress immunity, allowing cancers to grow faster. But I doubt that they play much of a role in their origin. Women with this disease did not "give themselves cancer" as a result of any sort of emotional failure.

How Safe Is Vitamin C?

Q:
Several months ago, the results of carefully planned and carried-out research on human subjects at the National Institutes of Health (NIH) suggested that the RDA for vitamin C should be increased to 200 milligrams a day. Daily intake of more than 800 or 1,000 milligrams may actually be harmful, according to the study. Why have you chosen to stick with your recommendation of 1,000 to 2,000 milligrams a day in the face of these findings?

A:
The doses I suggest are actually very modest doses, compared to those recommended by the ultimate vitamin C enthusiast, the late Linus Pauling. He took 18,000 milligrams of vitamin C a day.

I wouldn't go quite that far, but I do recommend 1,000 milligrams twice a day at minimum. We get vitamin C from fruits and vegetables, and we need more of it when exposed to toxins, infection, and chronic illness. If you eat an unhealthy diet or have increased cancer risks for any reason, I'd go up to 2,000 milligrams three times a day. The best form to take is a soluble powder, purchased in bulk (1/4 teaspoon equals 1,000 milligrams). I recommend a nonacidic form, because it's easier on your teeth and stomach. Avoid chewable tablets packed with sugar.

I've never seen any toxicity from vitamin C. The only problem that large doses commonly cause is bowel intolerance: flatulence and diarrhea. If this happens, you should just cut back to a more comfortable dose. You can also trigger a deficiency by taking large doses and then stopping suddenly, because the body gets lazy about absorbing it.

The NIH studied absorption of vitamin C into the blood, not its effects on immune function or its ability to counteract degenerative disease. The problem the researchers encountered in doses of about 1,000 milligrams had to do with high production of oxalate, which can spur kidney stones in some people. A magnesium supplement a day can help deter kidney stones, as does remembering to drink plenty of water.

There is one other caution. Recently, doctors have learned that rare individuals suffer from iron overload, usually the result of taking iron supplements or of liver disease. Vitamin C increases the absorption of iron, and high doses can cause serious problems for these individuals.

Some of the advantages of vitamin C, such as the strengthening of blood vessels and connective tissue, do not occur at the levels recommended by the NIH. High vitamin C intake has been linked to denser bones, lowered risk of heart attack, and alleviation of asthma. I don't view vitamin C as a cure for all illnesses, but I do believe we have yet to discover all of its benefits.

The U.S. government approaches setting recommended daily allowances from the perspective of preventing deficiency diseases like scurvy, so the numbers are going to be on the low end. I'm looking at vitamins quite differently—as natural therapeutic agents with a variety of beneficial effects—which is why I consistently recommend more than the RDAs.

Does Vitamin C Aid Recovery from Surgery?

Q:

Have you heard about the intravenous use of vitamin C both before and after surgery to promote faster healing?

A:

Yes. I usually recommend taking 20 grams of vitamin C a day mixed with intravenous fluids, beginning with the IV drip in the operating room and continuing for five days, or until the drip is removed. The problem? Many patients have their requests turned down, either by their doctor or by the hospital pharmacy staff, who are likely to say it's not part of their protocol. Persist. Have your family and friends persist. Say you'll go to another hospital. Then you should be able to get it done. Recently, a friend's brother had surgery for esophageal cancer, and his physician—one of the top gastric surgeons in New York—at first resisted his request for vitamin C, but eventually complied. The result was not surprising to me; the surgeon was so impressed with the speed of healing that he now plans to use vitamin C therapy with other patients.

Looking for Alternatives in Cancer Care?

Q:
Do you know of a reputable center for alternative cancer therapy?

A:
There is no one right treatment for cancer. And, unfortunately, there is no one magical alternative out there.

First, I'd determine just what sort of help is needed. Michael Lerner has written an excellent book, *Choice in Healing,* on integrating alternative and conventional treatments. As Lerner recommends, it's important to consider three factors: the plausibility of the therapy itself, the character of the practitioner, and the quality of service at the center. I would ask you to also consider the expense and practicality of going to any treatment center. An appendix in Lerner's book describes specific therapies and their better-known practitioners.

For cancers that are growing rapidly, the benefits of chemotherapy or radiation may outweigh the risks. If you decide to use the conventional therapies, then I would look for guidance on nutrition, dietary supplements, and mind-body techniques, all of which can increase their effectiveness and reduce their toxicity. Many of the alternative cancer centers use this approach.

If you decide not to use conventional therapies, then you'll need to shop around and evaluate success rates of other treatments. Some centers use therapies that are not accepted by the medical establishment, even though the centers may be staffed by M.D.s. I don't know that there's any one approach that has consistent success, although there are well-documented cases of individuals who have done well on alternative regimens.

Interesting practitioners include Dr. Nicholas Gonzalez in New York City and Dr. Stanislaw Burzynski in Houston, Texas, both of whom are M.D.s. Dr. Gonzalez is using an updated version of a complex nutritional therapy developed by the late William D. Kelley, a dentist from Texas. The treatment involves highly individualized diets; massive vitamin, mineral, and enzyme supplementation, and detoxification using coffee enemas. Dr. Burzynski focuses his work on antineoplastons, peptide molecules he discovered in human urine. There is considerable controversy over the effectiveness of his very expensive therapy. In fact, a recent case in federal court (brought by the government) sought to determine whether Burzynski was guilty of violating federal regulations in his use of an unapproved cancer treatment. It ended in a hung jury.

Treatments at many alternative cancer clinics are expensive, and, of course, insurance doesn't cover them. It's a good idea to see if the place you're considering will put you in touch with people who have been there. If they won't do that, I would be suspicious.

Consider especially what sort of success the practitioner may have had with the specific type of cancer you're dealing with. I'd also talk to other cancer specialists, and to nurses and other medical assistants who work in the clinic.

Crippled by Carpal Tunnel Syndrome?

Q:

Due to repetitive typing I have developed carpal tunnel syndrome in both arms. I was given anti-inflammatory medication for this. Then I developed stomach problems— gastritis and irritable bowel syndrome. I recently have begun to see a doctor of Eastern medicine, who started me on herbs including ginger tablets with DGL (deglycyrrhizinated licorice). On my second visit he performed acupuncture. Do you think that with Eastern medicine my carpal tunnel will also get better?

A:

When you're an especially speedy typist or spend long hours at the keyboard, the tendons that move the fingers can swell. There's one little tunnel through the ligament at the base of your palm that all the tendons and one very important nerve pass through from your arm to your hand. That's where the swelling can cause pressure and pain, the condition known as carpal tunnel syndrome (CTS).

The most effective treatment that I've found is vitamin B-6 (pyridoxine), 100 milligrams, two or three times a day. In this dosage, pyridoxine is not acting as a B vitamin but rather as a natural therapeutic agent that relieves nerve compression injuries. Be aware that doses of B-6 higher than 300 milligrams a day have caused rare cases of nerve damage. Discontinue usage if you develop any unusual numbness. (A much-publicized University of Michigan study warned about nerve toxicity with B-6 and discouraged people from using it for CTS. I disagree.)

For quick relief when you're hurting, rub on arnica gel, which you can find in your health food store or drugstore. Also, try wrapping ice packs around your wrists (a bag of frozen peas works just as well); if you use this treatment for five minutes every few hours when you're especially stressing your wrists, it may ease the pain and the inflammation. The ginger you mention may relieve inflammation over time, and acupuncture certainly can provide symptomatic relief.

The most important consideration when you've got CTS is to figure out ways to reduce the repetitive strain. Unless you do so, long-term improvement is unlikely. That means doing less typing, and learning how to stop driving yourself so hard at the keyboard. Here are a few other tips: Make yourself stand up every hour for a few minutes and stretch. The muscles in your wrists are connected to those in your arms, shoulders, and neck. Pay attention to those parts of your body, too, because stretching and relaxing your shoulders, neck, and back can ease the strain on your wrists. I know some people who have found relief through deep-tissue massage or Rolfing. And consider whether you're feeling emotional tension at work that can tighten your whole body, making it more susceptible to injury.

Your posture at the keyboard can make a big difference. Sit up straight, with your weight slightly forward. Your feet should be flat on the floor, or tilted comfortably on an adjustable footrest. An adjustable keyboard tray will allow you to change the position of your hands now and then, and keep your wrists straight, with your forearms horizontal and at a 90-degree angle to your upper arms. Your elbows should be at your sides in a relaxed position. Every now and then, tilt your head slowly to each side, and roll your shoulders twice forward and twice back. Squeeze your hands into tight fists, and then stretch your fingers out as wide as they will go. Close your hands into fists again and rotate your wrists a few times in either direction.

You might also try a different keyboard. Each brand has its own key touches and key widths, some of which may feel better to you than others. If you can find a split keyboard, it may help you keep your hands and arms at a more natural angle. There are also some new keyboards with concave keys, sections tilted up like an accordion, and other unusual shapes. I haven't tried them, but you may want to check them out.

Should Chemo and Antioxidants Be Mixed?

Q:

In your book Spontaneous Healing, *you advise discontinuing antioxidants during chemotherapy. My sister, who was diagnosed with ovarian cancer, is scheduled for eight chemo treatments three weeks apart over a twenty-four-week period. Should she discontinue antioxidants for the entire twenty-four weeks, or can she take them after each individual treatment? If so, how soon after each treatment can she start, and how soon before each treatment should she stop?*

A:

You're right. I wrote in *Spontaneous Healing* that "if you decide to proceed with radiation or chemotherapy, [you should] discontinue use of antioxidant supplements during treatment, since they may protect cancer cells along with normal cells." In general, antioxidants protect cells from damage by free radicals and other toxins. The safest antioxidants are vitamin C, vitamin E, selenium, and beta-carotene. Together, they block the chemical reactions that create free radicals, which can damage DNA and promote a variety of degenerative changes in cells. Chemotherapy and radiation generate free radicals; that is how they kill dividing cells. By taking antioxidants during chemotherapy, your sister would be reducing the effectiveness of the chemo treatment.

I would discontinue the antioxidants a few days before the start of chemotherapy and stay off them during the entire course of therapy. Then I think your sister could resume within two weeks of chemo-therapy. The same holds true with regard to radiation.

Once your sister is finished with chemotherapy, the antioxidants could be helpful. In fact, some studies in-dicate that antioxidants may help slow the growth of cancerous cells. In addition, cancer is a systemic dis-ease that should be approached from a whole-body perspective. Making a variety of changes to improve one's general health can be very important. Working to heal relationships, keeping up regular exercise, using tonic herbs with immune-enhancing effects, practicing visualization, and taking antioxidants can all help create an environment conducive to optimum health and healing.

By the way, your sister could take immune-protective herbs, such as astragalus, or extracts of reishi or maitake mushrooms during her treatment; they will not interfere with chemotherapy or radiation.

Care for Some Chicken Soup?

Q:
Is there anything to chicken soup as a cold remedy?

A:
Chicken soup. Just the mention of it conjures up images of steaming broth, packed with carrots, celery, peppercorns, and onion; chunks of chicken; maybe some noodles thrown in. How could it not be a good remedy?

It's comforting, it's warm, and it's fluid. At the University of Nebraska Medical Center, researchers found that chicken soup indeed had anti-inflammatory properties. They discovered that it reduced cold symptoms even when extremely diluted. Apparently the soup inhibits white blood cells called neutrophils, allowing them to fight infection without causing inflammation.

But chicken soup is more than just ingredients. It's comfort, love, and caring, captured in a mixture that fills your nose with fragrant steam and warms your insides. Much of chicken soup's curative power comes from its function as a placebo. (When something has a powerful effect because you believe it will, it's called a placebo.)

Of course, your relationship with chicken soup is affected by your cultural background. In some regions, fish soup is considered the universal elixir.

Whatever soup you choose, its benefits also stem from the love and caring it embodies—whether you make the soup yourself or someone gives it to you. It's clear that soup can be a natural remedy that helps you access your own natural healing power.

How to Treat Chlamydia?

Q:
A woman claims to have gotten chlamydia from me twice, in 1986 and 1989. I couldn't have given it to her, since I never had any symptoms. Pelvic inflammatory disease was diagnosed in her in 1986 and chlamydia in 1989. Tetracycline was prescribed to her both times. No M.D. ever asked to speak to me. Doctors have told me that chlamydia testing was extremely unreliable back then and as recently as 1992 was stopped at George Washington Medical Center because of high false positives and negatives. Is there any way to test now if I ever had it? Is there any record of test reliability in that time period? Would I have any noticeable symptoms if I had it? Any other comments?

A:
Chlamydia is the most common sexually transmitted disease, with an estimated 4 million infections from the organism occurring every year. The infection can cause serious problems in women, beginning with pelvic inflammatory disease and possibly leading to ectopic pregnancy or infertility. Almost three-quarters of women with the disease don't notice any symptoms, which can include vaginal discharge or painful urination.

Diagnosis of chlamydia is difficult, as you point

out, but some newer and more accurate diagnostic tests are available. Scientists at Johns Hopkins have developed a new urine test for chlamydia that is simpler, more convenient, and just as sensitive as older methods (taking small scrapings of cells from a woman's cervix or a swab from a man's urethra). The Hopkins test uses a technology called DNA amplification, which is like a super–copying machine for genes. By producing millions of copies of genetic material found in the *Chlamydia* organism, this test makes the disease more easily detectable in the laboratory. The Hopkins test is especially useful to determine if treatment has been successful.

There's certainly no way to test now whether you had it years ago. There's a high chance that chlamydia will be asymptomatic in men, which is one of the reasons it gets passed around so much. In fact, reported cases for women are more than five times as great as for men, in part because men are rarely tested for it.

When the symptoms do occur in men, they commonly include mildly painful urination and a scanty to moderate penile discharge. You probably should have received tetracycline in the same dose as your partner. Anytime one sex partner has chlamydia, the other one should be treated as well.

Finally, I think it's important to remember that both parties need to take responsibility for sexual health these days. I detect a tone in your question, implying that your woman friend was somehow at fault. Laying blame has no place in this discussion.

What's It Take to Lower Cholesterol?

Q:
*I have very high cholesterol that is obviously heredi-
tary since I'm a vegetarian and eat no animal products. I consume very little fat, and I take vitamin E. I
want to avoid medication. Is there anything I can take
in the way of herbs or natural products to lower my
cholesterol? And yes, I do exercise regularly.*

A:
I'm assuming from your question that you've done all
of the standard lifestyle interventions to try to ma-
nipulate cholesterol. The primary step, of course, is to
reduce saturated fat in your diet as much as possible,
meaning mostly fats of animal origin, but also palm
and coconut oils. Peanut butter, vegetable oils, short-
enings, and margarines can also cause your body to
make too much cholesterol. Also cut out coffee, black
tea, and cola.

On the positive side, Japanese green tea and foods
like onions, garlic, chili peppers, and shiitake mushrooms all have some cholesterol-lowering effects.
Also—as you know—make sure you exercise. (I always recommend thirty minutes, at least five days a
week.)

Most people find that changing their eating and exercise habits brings their cholesterol profile down to
normal. But everyone's biochemical balance is unique,

so these interventions may not have worked for you. If they haven't, then I think it may be time to try niacin, or vitamin B-3.

There have been some ineffective forms of niacin on the market. But there's a new form that definitely works, a wax-impregnated, time-release niacin tablet. J. R. Carlson Laboratories, based in Arlington Heights, Illinois, is one of the companies that make it, in a product called Niacin-Time. I would start with a dose of one 500-milligram tablet twice a day with meals.

I will caution you, though, to take niacin with great care and with medical supervision. Time-release niacin is very effective at lowering cholesterol, but it can also disturb liver function. In rare cases, it can cause a toxic fulminant hepatitis. That's a real medical catastrophe that can be fatal.

You must monitor liver function when starting time-release niacin. Have liver function checked at the start of therapy, then test it again after two weeks on niacin. You can get a liver test at any clinical laboratory, but a doctor has to phone in an order for it.

As long as your liver enzymes are normal you can stay on the niacin indefinitely, increasing the dose until cholesterol comes down to the level you want. You may want to go up to 1,500 milligrams a day or even higher, but I'll emphasize again that this can only be done with liver monitoring. Keep the dose as low as possible to maintain improvement. You should also know the early signs of liver dysfunction: unexplained loss of appetite, nausea, a feeling of abdominal fullness, abdominal pain, and any other unusual digestive symptoms.

Don't take niacin if you are pregnant or have ulcers,

gout, diabetes, gallbladder disease, or liver disease, or have had a recent heart attack.

Niacin seems to both lower the bad LDL (low-density lipoprotein) cholesterol, which damages artery walls, and maybe raise HDL (high-density lipoprotein), the good cholesterol that protects arteries. Your total cholesterol should be under 180. If you can get your total cholesterol under 150, your chance of a heart attack is negligible.

Chromium: Supplement of the Month?

Q:

I've been hearing a lot of talk lately about chromium, both on the news and from some friends in the health business. What exactly does it do, and do you feel it is a beneficial addition to a vitamin diet? Thanks!

A:

You're right, there's a lot of buzz about chromium these days, notably a recent report claiming that chromium produces "spectacular" results in normalizing glucose and insulin levels in adult-onset diabetes. The Department of Agriculture study recommended that diabetics take 1,000 micrograms a day.

There's also been a lot of promotion from the manufacturers of one form, chromium picolinate. I often see ads for this product that make unsubstantiated claims like this one:

DIET BOOSTER TABLETS
with Chromium Picolinate

3 STEP FAT ATTACK . . .
Appetite Suppressant to
reduce cravings for food.

Fat Metabolizer for efficient metabolic
breakdown of fats, carbs, and proteins.

Diuretic Action assists in
reducing excess fluids.

CHROMIUM PICOLINATE (200 micrograms)
A natural fat metabolizer. This form of
Chromium plays a vital role in the
functioning of insulin responsible for
regulating the efficient metabolism of fats,
carbohydrates, and protein.

These are megaclaims: that chromium will help you lose weight, stabilize blood sugar, treat hypoglycemia, lower cholesterol, and improve blood fats. Unless you're diabetic or deficient in chromium—and most people aren't deficient—I don't think supplemental chromium will do anything for you. This is another example of the supplement-of-the-month mentality that we're seeing all the time. We all want to take a pill to solve our problems, and the manufacturers are ready to sell it to us. Enough said.

Help for Chronic Fatigue Syndrome?

Q:

My wife has had chronic fatigue syndrome for the past six years. Traditional medicine has seemed to offer very little to her and in the past has actually made her worse. Many M.D.s, including many who specialize in the field, still seem not to have a clue about how to treat this illness. What suggestions do you have for overcoming this disease?

A:

Many people have written in about chronic fatigue syndrome (CFS), a condition known incorrectly as "chronic Epstein-Barr virus disease" or "chronic EBV." I'm not sure anybody knows exactly what chronic fatigue syndrome is; right now it appears to be a faddish disease that may or may not prove to be a true clinical entity. My suspicion is that if you look at a hundred people with the diagnosis, you might actually find many different conditions present—some purely emotional (such as depression) and others that might involve chronic viral infections.

The most important information I can give you is that the syndrome will end. Don't believe people who tell you otherwise.

I agree that conventional medicine has little to offer. Some doctors attempt treatment with injections of gamma globulin, interferon, or the antiviral drug acyclovir. These are pretty drastic methods that may do more harm than good. It sounds as though your wife has already been subjected to some of these treatments; generally I advise staying away from them.

Unfortunately, alternative practitioners often take advantage of patients with CFS and charge them a lot of money for treatments of questionable value.

Here are my general recommendations for people with CFS:

- Take astragalus root for its antiviral and immunity-enhancing properties. I've used Astra-8, a mixture of astragalus and seven other Chinese herbs. Take three tablets twice a day. You should have no problem staying on it indefinitely.
- Take maitake mushrooms, generally available in health food stores. These are nontoxic and may speed recovery. Follow dosage on the product container.
- Take my antioxidant formula (see page 10). In addition, take 60–100 milligrams of coenzyme Q, plus a B-100 B-complex supplement.
- Eat a low-protein, low-fat, high-carbohydrate diet.
- Eat one to two cloves of raw garlic a day. Garlic is a potent antibiotic, with antibacterial and antiviral effects as well. (By the way, a clove of garlic is one of the segments making up the head or bulb. Don't eat the whole bulb!) Chop it fine and mix with food, or swallow chunks like pills.
- Be careful about joining support groups. Find a

group that encourages recovery, not the idea that you will be sick forever.

Again, tell your wife not to despair. Many of my patients have recovered. I'd like to hear back from you in two to three months, after you've tried these methods.

Killing Me Softly with Your Cloves?

Q:

How bad for you are clove cigarettes compared to regular cigarettes? I've read conflicting reports and have heard that one clove cigarette is equivalent to smoking an entire pack of regular cigarettes. Please give me your advice.

A:

Sometimes people mistakenly assume that clove cigarettes are healthier than regular cigarettes because cloves are more "natural," but those people must not have read the labels. Clove cigarettes are just tobacco with clove flavor. That may mean tobacco mixed with cloves, but often it means tobacco mixed with artificial clove flavoring and other fragrances. Clove cigarettes are also usually unfiltered, and they may deliver three times as much tar as a regular Marlboro.

Still, I can't believe that smoking one clove cigarette is equivalent to smoking an entire pack of regular cigarettes. But clove cigarette smoke can be more irritating than the smoke of regular cigarettes, depending on individual sensitivity.

Everything we know regarding secondhand smoke and tobacco is applicable to clove cigarettes because of the tobacco in them. Plus, to me, the smoke smells worse than plain tobacco smoke. I'm not sure of all the health risks of inhaling components of clove oil on a regular basis, but there are reported cases of allergic pneumonitis (inflammation of the lungs) in people who smoke clove cigarettes.

What Do You Do with Coenzyme Q?

Q:
What is coenzyme Q and why do you take it?

A:
Coenzyme Q, also known as ubiquinone, is a natural substance found in most foods; it assists in oxygen utilization and energy production by cells, especially heart-muscle cells. Many medical papers demonstrate coenzyme Q's usefulness as a preventive as well as a treatment. In general, coenzymes work with enzymes to help them in their various biochemical functions. Coenzymes are smaller than proteins and so can survive digestion and pass into the system. Coenzyme Q was approved in Japan in 1974 to treat congestive heart failure and has also been approved in Sweden, Italy, Denmark, and Canada. Some people say coenzyme Q increases aerobic endurance, but more studies are needed to verify this. I often recommend it to help stabilize blood sugar in people who have diabetes and to strengthen the heart muscle. It also maintains the health of gums and other tissues. There is evidence that coenzyme Q can prolong survival in women with breast cancer, too.

Your body makes coenzyme Q, and you take it in when you eat fish, meats, and oils from soybean, sesame, and rapeseed (canola). The supplement form is imported from Japan. I take 100 milligrams once a day with food as a general health-booster. Co-enzyme Q is harmless, but it's not cheap.

Fighting a Cold?

Q:
I've spent too much money on all these fancy over-the-counter products for colds. Sometimes they mask the symptoms, but they don't really seem to make me better. Any other recommendations?

A:
You're absolutely right. Most of the over-the-counter products don't help you heal, even if they do stop the sniffles and headaches for a short while. I learned recently that more over-the-counter products are sold for the common cold than for any other disease. Not really surprising. Over the years, I have been collecting home remedies for colds—using myself and my family as guinea pigs. Here's what I've found works best:

Take vitamin C to prevent colds—2,000 milligrams, three times a day. You should start this now.

As soon as you start feeling cold symptoms, eat two cloves (not heads) of raw garlic. Trust me on this. You may not be kissing anyone soon, but garlic has powerful antibiotic effects. Chop it up and mix it with food, or swallow larger pieces like pills.

You can also take echinacea (*Echinacea purpurea* and related species) at the first sign of a cold or flu—like a scratchy throat or achy back. Take a dropperful of the tincture in a little warm water (or tea) four times a day. Use half doses for children.

Try sucking on zinc gluconate or zinc acetate lozenges, which, according to a recent study, may cut the duration of a cold in half.

Finally, drink this powerful gingerroot tea for head and chest congestion, malaise, and the chills. Here's my recipe:

Grate a 1-inch piece of peeled gingerroot. Put it in a pot with 2 cups of cold water, bring to a boil, lower heat, and simmer five minutes. Add $1/2$ teaspoon cayenne pepper (or more or less to taste) and simmer one minute more. Remove from heat. Add 2 tablespoons of fresh lemon juice, honey to taste, and 1 or 2 cloves of mashed garlic. Let cool slightly, and strain if you desire.

Then get under the covers and drink as much of it as you like. Hope you feel better.

Charmed by
Colloidal Minerals?

Q:
How do you feel about taking colloidal mineral supplements?

A:
To me these supplements exemplify obnoxious, multi-level marketing in the name of natural medicine. I've received countless copies of an audiotape that advertises colloidal minerals and makes all sorts of unsubstantiated claims. The veterinarian who pitches the stuff is said to have been nominated for the Nobel Prize in medicine. Well, anyone can write a letter to the Nobel Prize committee. I could nominate you for the Nobel Prize in medicine. I have not seen convincing evidence of therapeutic benefit from taking colloidal minerals. And these products may deliver some substances you definitely don't need—aluminum, for example.

Well, I feel better after venting.

"Colloidal" means the mineral particles are of a certain size, facilitating use by the body. The marketers will tell you that their products make you live twice as long, protect you from cancer, and cure just about anything. They'll tell you that mineral deficiencies lead to a weakened immune system and cancer. You can buy the products as liquid supplements, aerosols, injectables, and vaginal douches. The literature in health food stores says they're powerful anti-microbials and immune-system stimulants; they're supposed to help cure as many as 650 different diseases. None of these claims are proven.

Some colloidal minerals have a long history as medicinals. In the nineteenth century, for example, colloidal silver was promoted as a treatment for everything from colds to rheumatism. Silver products are useful as germicides, but over time they've been replaced by safer and more effective ones.

There is some potential for harm as well. The body doesn't need silver, and the mineral can accumulate in tissues, causing an irreversible bluish discoloration of the skin. There are even some reports of neurological problems in people who have used oral silver products long-term.

Bottom line: I don't recommend colloidal minerals; there's no reason to think they're as good for you as they are for their marketers. Besides, you should be getting your minerals in highly usable form from fruits and vegetables in your diet. Please eat more fruits and vegetables—organically grown, when possible.

Expired Contact Lenses?

Q:

Why do my disposable contact lenses have an expiration date? Is it dangerous to wear them beyond that date?

A:

It's really important to follow manufacturers' instructions about contact lenses. That thin piece of plastic that helps you see sits directly on your eye. About half the 18.2 million contact lens wearers in the United States use soft lenses, which are especially likely to cause infection if special handling techniques aren't followed. The plastic can become brittle over time, and the lenses can become carriers for bacteria. You should return or throw away lenses that have expired.

Two organisms, *Pseudomonas aeruginosa* and *Acanthamoeba castellanii,* are especially associated with infections of the cornea from poor contact lens hygiene. People like you who wear disposable lenses are at highest risk for infection. In one study, people who used disposable daily-wear lenses had a 49 percent higher risk of *Acanthamoeba* infection than those who wore conventional soft lenses. The most common reasons for infection were failure to disinfect the lenses and use of chlorine-release lens disinfection systems, which aren't effective against that particular organism.

Even if you wear lenses approved for overnight wear, don't keep them on overnight. With that kind of usage, there is a much greater chance of damaging the cornea and allowing bacteria to build up.

Going Crazy
with Crabs?

Q:
Could crab lice be transmitted in the steam room of a gym? I assure you, I have not had sexual activity for the past six months. Somehow, I got crabs and I am embarrassed to go to my doctor. He probably won't believe me.

A:
First of all, never let embarrassment stop you from going to a doctor. It's part of his or her job not to make judgments, and besides, doctors have seen it all. I know! If your doctor makes you feel ashamed, then you're going to the wrong doctor.

Sexual contact is the most common method of transmitting crabs, but there are plenty of other modes. You can get crabs from sharing the clothing, bedding, or towels of an infested person. However, the temperature in the steam room would make it difficult for the lice to survive and hop from one person to another, so, frankly, I think you must have gotten them from another source.

Many years ago, a friend of mine told me that he once had a houseguest who shared towels with everyone in the house (a married couple and their three teenage children included). Unfortunately, the guest had crabs, and soon, so did everyone else in the house. Very quietly a "health emergency" was proclaimed, treatment and cleaning were begun, and the house-guest was sent away. I wonder what Miss Manners would have to say about that!

Crab lice get their name because they look very much like miniature crabs. Once on the body, they cling between two hairs, bury their heads underneath the skin, and feed on blood. They attach their tiny white eggs to hairs. The biting and moving around makes for severe itching and irritation. It doesn't take very many crabs to cause great discomfort. And they multiply very quickly.

You can get rid of crab lice just as you would head lice. One popular preparation is Kwell, which is 1 percent lindane, but it's toxic to people as well as lice. Lindane, a cousin of DDT, is easily absorbed into the skin and can affect the central nervous system. You're better off using a pyrethrin insecticide, a natural insecticide from chrysanthemums. Neem, made from a tree in India, is another natural alternative. You can find them in garden stores.

Or use a treatment recommended by Kathi Keville in *Herbs for Health and Healing,* adapted for the pubic area:

> 2 ounces vegetable oil
> 20 drops tea tree essential oil
> 10 drops each, essential oils of rosemary, lavender, and lemon

Combine ingredients and first test them on the inside of your elbow for several hours. If there is no sign of irritation, then apply the treatment to your dry pubic hair. Cover the area with plastic wrap, followed by a towel. Leave these coverings on for one hour. Then work shampoo into the hair to cut the oil, rinse, and shampoo and rinse again. You'll probably need to do this a week later to get rid of any newly hatched lice.

And don't forget to clean all your towels, bed linens, and infested clothing. You don't want to become reinfested.

Cursing Your Cramps?

Q:
Is there any other way to stop cramps while having my period—other than with painkillers?

A:
Two-thirds of all women suffer from menstrual cramps. Until a couple of decades ago, the pain they endured was written off as a psychological "female problem" that women created for themselves. But in the late 1970s, researchers discovered a hormone called prostaglandin F_2 alpha that is released as the uterine lining breaks down, causing the uterus to go into spasm and hurt.

You can moderate the release of PGF_2 alpha through some dietary measures, primarily a low-fat, high-complex carbohydrate diet. Don't eat dairy products, and ease up on the meat and eggs. Cut back on fried foods and commercially baked foods. Most important, make sure you get enough essential fatty acids. If you have plenty of essential fatty acids in your system, your body will produce less PGF_2 alpha and more of a different hormone that helps prevent cramps. In one study, women who took 1.8 grams of omega-3 fatty acids in fish-oil capsules twice a day for two months had a significant improvement in cramps, nausea, and headaches. They used half as much aspirin as they had previously. I know other women who say oil of evening primrose works wonderfully for the same purpose, at a dose of two to three 500-milligram capsules twice a day.

In *Women's Bodies, Women's Wisdom,* Christiane Northrup, M.D., recommends a series of supplements to protect against cramps: 100 milligrams of vitamin B-6 per day, 50 IU of vitamin E (in the form of d-alpha-tocopherol) three times a day, and 100 milligrams of magnesium three to four times a day. While you're menstruating, she suggests 100 milligrams of magnesium every two hours to ease pain.

There are some effective traditional remedies for cramps as well, such as raspberry leaf tea. It's non-toxic, so you can consume as much as you like. An herb called cramp bark (*Viburnum opulus*), from a European bush, is a stronger remedy. The dose is one dropperful of the tincture in warm water as needed.

I'd also try acupuncture. There are pressure points that some people say will help, such as the acupuncture point on the wrist that's used for alleviating nausea, or a point on the inside of the foot that's used by reflexologists.

Smoking has been linked to added menstrual pain. And remember how much of an influence stress can be. Try to reduce stress in your life and practice relaxation techniques, such as meditation or yoga.

Is Decaf Really Any Better?

Q:

How much safer is decaf than regular coffee?

A:

Although new caffeine extraction methods seem to preserve the flavor of a good cup of coffee, decaffeinated coffee is not necessarily the answer for java junkies. Decaf retains enough caffeine to affect sensitive individuals. It also contains other substances naturally found in the coffee bean that can have irritating effects on the body. For example, decaffeinated coffee can be just as rough on the stomach as regular coffee.

If you have reason to avoid coffee, you would do well to avoid decaf also. If you have any of the following conditions, stay away from both drinks: migraine, tremor, anxiety, irregular heartbeat, insomnia, coronary heart disease or a strong family history of it, high cholesterol, any gastrointestinal disorder, any urinary disorder, prostate trouble, fibrocystic breasts, premenstrual syndrome, tension headaches, or seizure disorder.

A study done at the University of California at Berkeley found a relationship between drinking decaf and a slightly increased risk of high cholesterol and heart disease. In that survey of about 45,500 men, regular coffee did not have the same effect.

If you really want to drink decaf, I'd recommend using only the water-extracted versions. There is concern that traces of solvents may remain in coffee decaffeinated by other methods, although the manufacturers deny it.

There are many coffee substitutes available in supermarkets and health food stores. They are made from roasted grains, roots, acorns, and other benign ingredients. I recommend Cafix, Roma, Dacopa, and Teccino. Experiment with them, or use a caffeine-free herbal tea.

Does Deodorant Cause Breast Cancer?

Q:
Given that the sweat glands of the armpits are in close proximity to the breasts, has any research ever been done to see whether the use of deodorants has a positive correlation to the incidence of breast cancer in women?

A:
I'm not aware of any research on that topic. However, deodorants containing antiperspirants commonly cause inflammation of sweat glands and the formation of cysts under the arm. I would say this is reason enough not to use them.

The active ingredients in antiperspirant deodorants are aluminum compounds, which are irritants and may be absorbed into the body. We don't know the details of aluminum toxicity, but I recommend against exposing your tissues to this metal. Try natural forms of deodorants available in health food stores (the best ones contain extracts of green tea), or just splash rubbing alcohol under your arms as an antibacterial agent.

Fight Depression Without Drugs?

Q:
What alternatives are there to conventional anti-depressant medications or EST (electroshock therapy)? I have tried every medical therapy possible—except EST—but still face recurrent spontaneous episodes of major depression. Are there any alternative treatments that might halt this escalating cycle?

A:
There are only two alternative treatments for depression that I have any confidence in. The first is regular aerobic exercise, which can definitely provide a long-term solution. You'll have to do at least thirty minutes of some vigorous aerobic activity at least five times a week, and be prepared to wait several weeks before you see any benefit. Aerobic exercise is a preventive as well as a treatment.

The second is an herbal treatment called Saint-John's-wort (*Hypericum perforatum*). Saint-John's-wort is much used in Germany for the treatment of mild to moderate depression, as well as associated disturbed sleep cycles. Take 300 milligrams, three times a day, of a standardized extract containing at least 0.125 percent hypericin. Again, be prepared to wait two months before you see the full benefit.

Changes in your diet may also make a difference.

Try eating less protein and fat, and more starches, fruits, and vegetables. Experiment with the following amino acid and vitamin formula, for which you can find all the ingredients in a health food store. First thing in the morning, take 1,500 milligrams of DL-phenylalanine (DLPA, an amino acid), 100 milligrams of vitamin B-6, and 500 milligrams of vitamin C, along with a piece of fruit or a small glass of juice. Don't eat again for at least an hour. (DLPA can worsen high blood pressure, so use the formula cautiously if you have this condition, and start with a dose of 100 milligrams while monitoring your blood pressure.) Take another 100 milligrams of B-6 and more vitamin C in the evening.

You say you've taken a variety of drugs for depression. In general, I think that the new generation of antidepressants, including Prozac, Zoloft, and Paxil, are less toxic and more effective than medications of the past. Collectively known as SSRIs, or selective serotonin-reuptake inhibitors, they interact with the regulating mechanism for the neurotransmitter serotonin in your brain. It's best to be cautious with any of these drugs, particularly because their makers would have you believe that no one can live a normal life without them.

Make sure you aren't taking any other medications that may contribute to depression. These include antihistamines, tranquilizers, sleeping pills, and narcotics. Recreational drugs, alcohol, and coffee can also make depression worse.

You make reference to EST—electroshock or electroconvulsive therapy. That is a last resort for the treatment of severe depression. It does work, but I hope things won't get to the point where that's your only option.

Psychiatrists tend to look at all mental problems as stemming from disordered brain chemistry, hence their emphasis on drugs. I believe that disordered moods could just as easily lead to biochemical changes in the brain, so I look elsewhere for treatments. Buddhist psychology views depression as the necessary consequence of seeking stimulation. It counsels us to cultivate emotional balance in life, rather than always seeking highs and then regretting the lows that follow. The prescription is daily meditation, and I agree this may be the best way to get at the root of depression and change it.

Does DHEA Improve Memory?

Q:
My father-in-law takes DHEA along with a few other drugs, all under a doctor's care. He was having trouble remembering things and even being able to carry on a conversation. He says DHEA helps a lot, although he doesn't think it is enhancing his memory. What does DHEA do, exactly?

A:
DHEA is a natural hormone produced by the adrenal glands, in the family of male sex hormones. Currently there is great medical interest in DHEA (dehydro-epiandrosterone), as well as a push from the supplement industry to promote it as an antiaging, antiobesity, anticancer remedy. Smart-drug enthusiasts think it can also protect brain cells from the degenerative changes of old age. A lot of claims, but not a lot of conclusive science yet.

What we do know is that DHEA has a significant anabolic effect, which results in stronger bones and muscles and decreased body fat. It may protect health in a variety of ways. I've seen good results with DHEA in patients with autoimmune diseases like lupus. I also think it might help people with other diseases, such as asthma and rheumatoid arthritis, who have become dependent on prednisone, since it may allow them to wean their bodies off that more dangerous hormone. DHEA is sold as a prescription drug and by several mail-order pharmacies. Health food stores sell DHEA precursors, but those may be worthless. The extracts from wild yams will have no effect, either.

People who tout DHEA point out that we produce most of this hormone in our twenties, with production tapering off in our later years until we produce only about one-fifth as much. They suggest that supplemental DHEA beginning at age forty or fifty could improve quality of life. But evidence for DHEA's benefits is inconclusive. There was one small, six-month study at the University of California–San Diego that reported improved energy and feelings of well-being.

I'm cautious about using any hormones on a regular basis without good reason and without medical supervision. We don't know what the downside of taking supplemental DHEA may be over time. Ray Sahelian, M.D., author of *DHEA: A Practical Guide,* warns against taking high doses cavalierly and suggests consulting with a physician before trying DHEA, because it is a steroid that the body converts into potent estrogens and androgens. Side effects can include acne, facial hair growth in women, deepening of the voice, and mood changes. DHEA probably increases risk of prostate cancer and may increase risk of coronary heart disease.

If your father-in-law's chief concern is his memory, I would suggest an herbal preparation made from the leaves of the ginkgo tree (*Ginkgo biloba*). Researchers have recently begun to study the ability of ginkgo extracts to increase blood flow to the brain. You can buy this nontoxic product in any health food store. Your father-in-law could try taking two tablets or capsules three times a day with meals for memory enhancement. He might not notice any beneficial effects until he has used ginkgo for six to eight weeks.

Doubt the Need to Douche?

Q:

My doctor says this is a growing problem among women: Advertisers try very hard to make women feel unclean so they will buy their products. Douching washes away certain forms of bacteria that protect women from getting infections. When the bacteria aren't there, a woman's body becomes more vulnerable. I'd like to hear your opinion on this.

A:

Douching used to be conventional wisdom, but it's not anymore. Now medical opinion generally discourages women from douching. And when the concern is about hygiene or odor, the risks of douching are much greater than the benefits. Douching can change the pH (or acidity level) of your vagina to be less friendly to helpful bacteria and more attractive to the harmful ones. It can wash away protective flora and leave the tissues more likely to get inflamed or infected.

In her book *Women's Bodies, Women's Wisdom*, Christiane Northrup, M.D., comments on the way women are taught to believe that the vagina is offensive, requiring deodorants and special sanitization. She says about one-third of all women douche regularly, even though it can cause harm.

There are times, however, that douching can be useful in the short term. For instance, I often recommend douching with acidophilus or diluted tea tree oil for a vaginal infection. You can insert acidophilus culture directly into your vagina in capsule or liquid form. It's a "friendly" organism that will keep overaggressive populations of yeast at bay. Tea tree oil is a powerful germicide. Mix about 1½ tablespoons in a cup of warm water to treat yeast infections. Some women are sensitive to this substance; discontinue it at once if you notice any irritation or burning.

Douching also may sometimes serve a protective function. Ejaculation of semen increases the pH of the vagina for eight hours. If you've had intercourse with ejaculation at least three times in a twenty-four-hour period, it will change the pH of the vagina throughout that time and produce conditions more likely for certain bacteria to grow. A douche with 1 tablespoon of white vinegar per quart of warm water will help prevent problems.

E. coli in the Apple Juice?

Q:
I'm worried about drinking E. coli–*infected apple juice. How does this happen? What can I do to protect myself from* E. coli? *What are the symptoms—and remedies?*

A:
You are right to be worried. A 1996 outbreak of *E. coli* poisoning from Odwalla Company apple juice focused attention on the dangers of unpasteurized juice—a product we thought was as wholesome as apple pie. This outbreak came just weeks after a similar one in Connecticut, where 10 people were made ill by unpasteurized apple cider. In both cases, it appears that the juice manufacturers followed all recommended guidelines that apples be brushed and washed before being pressed into juice.

"*E. coli*" is an abbreviation for *Escherichia coli* bacteria—a mostly harmless germ that lives in the intestines of humans and animals; it helps its hosts by suppressing the growth of harmful bacteria and by synthesizing important vitamins. But in recent years, a virulent strain known as *E. coli* 0157:H7 has made headlines in a number of food-poisoning outbreaks around the world. This latest outbreak, traced to California apples, was small compared to other episodes.

In 1993, undercooked, fecally contaminated hamburgers from Jack-in-the Box killed 4 people and sickened some 700 others. In 1996 in Japan, more than 9,000 people were sickened by a similar strain. *E. coli*–infected apple juice was never considered a real possibility until a 1991 outbreak was traced to cider pressed in Massachusetts. According to the FDA, *E. coli* 0157:H7 is evolving and "has adapted to survive in a more acidic environment," such as unpasteurized apple cider.

E. coli infection occurs primarily in two ways. Bacteria can leak from animals' intestines into meat intended for human consumption. Or *E. coli* can be present in completely uncooked foods, such as juice. Illness from *E. coli* has also been traced to consumption of salami, deli roast beef, raw milk, lake water, mayonnaise, cantaloupe, and leafy vegetables like lettuce.

Infection often causes stomach cramps and bloody diarrhea several hours to several days after ingestion. There may be slight fever and possibly vomiting. Generally, the illness resolves in five to ten days, but in children under five and the elderly, the infection can cause hemolytic uremia syndrome (HUS), in which red blood cells are destroyed and the kidneys fail. This complication occurs in 2 to 7 percent of cases and can be fatal.

With juice, it's always difficult to pinpoint the source of contamination. Often apple juice is made from "ground-fall" or "drop" apples. When that juice is unpasteurized, any contaminants from the manure of grazing cows or deer—or from farm runoff—that are not completely washed off can get into the juice during pressing. Federal authorities are considering new requirements that juice shipped interstate be pasteurized. An alternative would be to test juice for the presence of *E. coli*.

If you're concerned, you can bring unpasteurized juice to a rolling boil, which will kill any lingering microorganisms. To protect yourself from *E. coli* infection from meat, wash your hands and all cutting surfaces thoroughly after handling raw meat, and be sure to cook meat to 160°.

As for treatment, there is little evidence that antibiotics help (they may increase risk of kidney complications). Anti-diarrheal agents should also be avoided. Time is usually the best treatment. HUS, however, is life-threatening, requiring intensive care in a hospital. If you have any reason to suspect you've ingested contaminated juice (or other foods) and are having symptoms, call your doctor or local health department.

Does Echinacea Fight Colds?

Q:

Is echinacea helpful in the treatment of colds and flu? Does it really work as an immune system "booster" to help protect against them? What is the proper dosage? Is it the same for treatment as for prevention? What parts of the plant should be used?

A:

Echinacea is a common plant in North America, cultivated ornamentally in gardens as purple coneflower. Besides being pretty, it really does work as an immune system booster. Echinacea is very popular as a medicinal, and there are hundreds of products made from it.

There is a great deal of research from Germany showing that echinacea increases the number and activity of key white blood cells involved in immunity. It is known to boost the activity of T cells and natural killer cells and the production of interferon. The herb is versatile and very safe. Take it at the first sign of a cold or flu—symptoms like a scratchy throat or achy back.

The root contains the highest concentration of echinacea's active material, although the leaves are also potent. Some products are made from the whole plant; I prefer tinctures made from the root. At the first sign of a cold or flu, take a dropperful of the tincture in a little warm water (or tea) four times a day. Use half that much for children. Make sure the echinacea is potent by putting a bit on your tongue; if it produces a marked numbing sensation after a few minutes, it's good.

I generally don't use echinacea as a preventive, though some people do. The only time I might is if I go on a long plane flight, where the air is recirculated and unhealthy. Then I take echinacea for a couple of days beforehand. To build immunity, you may want to try echinacea at half the adult dosage and stay on it for a while.

There's a popular belief among herbalists that echinacea loses its effectiveness if it's taken continually for more than two or three weeks. But there is no evidence to support that belief, so I think you can go on taking it for as long as you think you need it.

Truth About Endometriosis?

Q:

What special recommendations would you make regarding diet for endometriosis sufferers? Do you think this is an autoimmune disease?

A:

I don't know what the root cause of endometriosis is. Nobody does. It's a poorly understood disease, and the treatments are only partly helpful. The symptoms can be debilitating or just very bothersome: severe cramping, painful menstruation, intestinal problems, and sometimes depression. The condition is characterized by tissue that looks and behaves just like the lining of the uterus (endometrium), but grows elsewhere in the body: the abdominal cavity, the intestines, the ovaries, or the abdominal wall. And just like the lining of the uterus, this tissue builds up with hormonal changes over the month, then breaks down and bleeds. Blood in the abdomen causes intense inflammation that can be very painful. In some women, the result is severe scarring and organ dysfunction. Endometriosis is often associated with infertility, but hasn't been shown to cause it directly.

Endometriosis doesn't necessarily progress to damage within the pelvis, or contribute to infertility. Sometimes it's very hard to find it in the body, and more and more, doctors are learning that it's quite common, with as many as half of menstruating women living with it. So experts now believe that mild endometriosis may actually be normal, and not need any treatment. In fact, studies have found that in many instances it doesn't spread and grow worse over time at all.

The most popular theory about endometriosis rests on the idea that menstrual flow sometimes moves backwards and up through the fallopian tubes, then out into areas within the pelvis. There, the discarded tissue seems to implant and begin to grow. The hypothesis you mention is one of the most recent—that the immune system is misbehaving, failing to kill off stray endometrial cells and then pumping up their growth. Women with painful endometriosis often make antibodies against their own tissue, the hallmark of autoimmunity.

It's commonly held that pregnancy will protect against endometriosis, but recent studies have found no difference in incidence between women who have been pregnant and those who have not. It is clear that the condition is strongly affected by hormones, and hormone therapy is the favored treatment. I'd suggest minimizing your intake of estrogen from outside sources, such as commercially raised animal foods. Eat soy foods such as tofu, tempeh, and miso, which are rich in plant estrogens that can block more harmful forms of estrogen. Reduce the fat in your diet. Limit your alcohol intake. Make sure you get nourishing food and eat lots of fiber. Exercise regularly. Also, cut dairy foods from your diet. Try all this for one month and see whether it reduces the pain.

Stress will worsen this condition. Visualization,

hypnotherapy, and Chinese medicine can all be helpful. You may want to consult with an herbalist as well. Dr. Christiane Northrup has an excellent chapter on endometriosis in *Women's Bodies, Women's Wisdom*. She suggests taking a multivitamin with plenty of B-complex and magnesium (about 50 milligrams of each of the B vitamins and 400 to 800 milligrams of magnesium), in addition to maintaining a low-fat, high-fiber diet.

Could I Really
Use an Enema?

Q:

I read your book Spontaneous Healing *and found it absolutely marvelous. I was, however, surprised that you never mentioned enemas or colonics as an adjunctive therapy for detoxification. I know the Gerson therapy and other alternative cancer treatments make extensive use of these measures. What is your opinion about them?*

A:

Enemas enjoyed great popularity in the seventeenth and eighteenth centuries, when they were considered both fashionable and medically necessary. Louis XIV of France was quite an enthusiast, sometimes undergoing as many as four a day—often during meetings with dignitaries. At that time, people believed that constipation resulted from "hypochondriacal melancholy," a problem that afflicted only the most noble and intelligent men. Similar symptoms in women were associated with "hysteria," in which the overheated womb wandered through the body longing for fulfillment. Mayan shamans took hallucinogenic enemas; made with mead, tobacco juice, mushrooms, and morning glory seeds, the enemas must have induced massively altered states of consciousness.

Proponents of enemas today argue that they clean

away microorganisms, impacted feces, and dead cells while relieving constipation, backache, fatigue, headache, loss of concentration, and other maladies. Quite a list. Colonic irrigation involves flushing the entire colon with running water.

The Gerson therapy you mention uses coffee enemas, plus a special juice diet, as a treatment for cancer. Its purpose is to detoxify the body and restore normal function to poisoned cells, which then mobilize to fight tumors. Coffee by this route is stimulating and addictive, claims of enthusiasts notwithstanding. Whether coffee enemas really detoxify the liver or any other organ is an open question. I don't think there is any health need for enemas and colonics, despite their interesting history. The best way to ensure the health and normal cleanliness of the colon is to make sure you're having regular eliminations: eat a diet that's high in fiber, drink enough water, and get adequate exercise. Avoid putting things into you that are toxic in the first place. The colon sheds its entire lining and regenerates it every day, so it's impossible for anything to build up on its walls.

To increase your fiber intake, you can eat psyllium seed husks in a variety of forms. There's also an herbal bowel-regulator called Triphala, from the Ayurvedic tradition, that is very effective. You can get it from a health food store; follow the dosage recommendations on the label.

A short "fruit fast" can give your digestive system a rest. I've done a ten-day regimen that included two days of fresh fruit, two days of fruit juice, two days of water only, then two days of fruit juice, and finally two days of fruit. All along, I took a tablespoonful of powdered psyllium seed husks stirred into a big glass of water every day to give the intestines bulk.

Enemas and colonics are trendy, in part because there is an element of pleasure in them. That's fine as long as people are honest about it. You can become addicted to the sensation of colonics, and doing them addictively is not healthy. There's some risk of getting hepatitis or a perforated colon from them, but I think it's pretty small.

To Fast or Not to Fast to Lose Weight?

Q:

Is fasting an effective diet tactic? What are the best method and duration for a fast? What other sorts of health benefits or detriments are involved?

A:

Fasting is absolutely not an effective diet tool, because it will alter your metabolism in a direction that actually makes it harder to shed pounds. Most people, when they go back to eating, compensate by upping their consumption of calories.

There are benefits to fasting for purposes other than weight loss. (By fasting, I mean taking in nothing other than water or herbal teas. Restricting yourself to fruits, fruit juices, or other liquids can be helpful, but not in exactly the same way as fasting.) I have experimented with fasting one day a week and find it a useful physical and psychological discipline. I experience mental clarity and increased energy after a short-term fast.

Short-term fasting—up to three days—is a good home remedy for colds, flus, and toxic conditions. Combine it with rest and good mental states. Drink plenty of water to help flush out your system, and remember to stay warm and conserve your energy. Break your fast with light, plain foods.

Long-term fasting—more than three days—can

also be beneficial, but it is potentially dangerous, so do not attempt it without expert supervision. It is a drastic technique. I know people who have fasted from one to three months and achieved complete remission of diseases that resisted all other treatments (bronchial asthma, rheumatoid arthritis, ulcerative colitis). Unfortunately, the diseases often return when eating resumes.

Trawling for Help on Fish Oil

Q:
We've heard such varied opinions on fish-oil supplements that we want your opinion. Help!

A:
Fish oil is probably the most important dietary source of omega-3 fatty acids, which are vital nutrients. These fatty acids reduce inflammation, protect against the abnormal clotting associated with heart attacks, inhibit cancer, and protect brain function. There may be other benefits, too: a 1992 study published in the journal *Lancet,* for example, suggested that omega-3 fatty acids prolong pregnancy by a few days and improve birthweights.

However, I don't recommend that people take fish-oil supplements to reap the benefits of omega-3s. The oils used for commercial capsules may have toxic contaminants. Also, it's not clear that the isolated fish oils reproduce the benefits of actually eating fish.

It would be much better to eat two to three servings a week of fish that contain omega-3 fatty acids. These are the oily fish from cold northern waters: sardines, herring, mackerel, and wild salmon, which has more omega-3s than farmed salmon.

If you are vegetarian or don't like fish, the best source of omega-3s is flaxseed. You can buy the whole seeds very cheaply in health food stores, or you can order packages of golden flax seeds (with a grinder) from Heintzman Farms (see Other Resources, page 274). Keep them in the refrigerator, and grind a half cup or so at a time in a blender or coffee grinder. Sprinkle a tablespoonful of the resulting meal onto salads, baked potatoes, or cereals. As a daily supplement, this will give you plenty of omega-3s. And it tastes good: sweet and nutty.

Be aware that flax has a very high fiber content, so it can increase stool bulk and have a laxative effect. Most people find this welcome.

Desperately Seeking Relief from Fleas?

Q:
I'm desperately seeking relief from flea bites and the allergic reaction I get. I have tried numerous internal and external repellents (vitamin B-12, eucalyptus, pennyroyal) to no avail. The fleas find me, bite, and cause severe itching over my entire body. This is extremely uncomfortable and upsetting as they are leaving chicken pox–like scarring that lasts for months. Have you any experience with this?

A:
This is a tough one. Fleas love the humid conditions of Hawaii, coastal California, the Gulf Coast, and the Atlantic seaboard south of Maryland. Breeding conditions there are perfect year-round, and with one hundred fleas able to produce a half-million offspring in one month, you can see why they continue to find you.

I'm sorry to say your best hope may be to fumigate your house with chemical "bombs" available at pet food stores and veterinarians' offices. (Make sure you stay out of your house during the bombing process.) In my experience, the natural repellents that you mention don't work nearly as well as chemical pesticides for severe infestations.

Pyrethrins, active insecticidal agents found in flowers related to chrysanthemums, will kill the fleas and degrade rapidly in the environment. They are nontoxic to humans. You will need to use these or other treatments more than once in order to kill more than one generation of fleas. Growth regulators like fenoxycarb mimic flea hormones and prevent the young larvae from becoming adult fleas.

Another natural product you might try is called Neem. It's a powerful and relatively safe insecticide obtained from a tree in India. You should be able to find it at garden stores. Also, some people dust carpets, furniture, and the crevices where fleas hide out with diatomaceous earth, which contains the fossilized "skeletons" of sea algae. Organic farmers often use it to kill insects; its sharp crystals puncture their bodies.

There are biological insecticides that you can try outdoors. Several brands available at lawn and garden stores employ nematodes—tiny worms—that feed on the flea larvae.

You don't say whether you have pets. If you do, try keeping them outside the house. Wash their bedding in hot water and detergent and keep doing so once a week. Also, there's a relatively new product available from vets called Program, which you administer to your pet once a month. Many people have seen dramatic improvement in bad flea situations after starting to use Program.

Once you get things under control, vacuuming every other day may help remove the eggs that fleas lay in the carpet. Get rid of the vacuum bag each time, because the fleas will hatch inside. When you wash the floor, pay special attention to baseboards and areas under the furniture. Shampoo your carpets or bring in a professional steam cleaner at least twice a year. The best way to fight fleas is to keep your environment scrupulously clean.

To Fluoridate or Not?

Q:
My town is going to put fluoride in our drinking water. I don't feel good about this. What do you think?

A:
I'm aware of all the arguments for and against fluoride, and I can only conclude that this is primarily an emotional issue that does not lend itself to rational discussion. I've heard everything from concerns that it may cause bone cancer to the complaint that it's a government plot to destroy people's brains.

More than half the drinking water in this country is fluoridated (meaning small amounts of fluoride are added in order to strengthen teeth and reduce cavities). There are data supporting this use; a study in the late 1980s concluded that cavities decreased by 25 percent among children in communities with fluoridated water.

You don't want more than 2 parts per million of fluoride in your drinking water, however. More than that can cause chronic, low-level fluoride poisoning, especially since many people are also using dental products that contain fluoride. If your water is fluoridated, don't use more than a pea-sized bit of any fluoride toothpaste on your brush. Too much of this element may make your teeth mottled and chalky white in places, a condition known as fluorosis (this condition afflicts mostly children).

Great excesses of fluoride can cause weight loss, brittle bones, anemia, and weakness. And some data do suggest increased cancer risk. All in all, the scientific information is contradictory, fueling the controversy rather than settling it. For example, some studies indicate that fluoridation of water contributes to hip fractures in older men and women, but other studies show no such effect.

If you're concerned about fluoride in your drinking water, filter it out. You can do this by using any of the water purifying systems—reverse osmosis and distillation, for example—that remove minerals (see page 273). If you decide to do this, however, I'd recommend that you give growing children supplemental fluoride to protect their teeth. Talk to your dentist for help with that.

Obviously, overdoses of fluoride are toxic. But in low doses, I believe, the benefits for children's teeth are immeasurable.

Getting Enough Folic Acid?

Q:
How important is folic acid? Can't I get this and other B vitamins in a balanced diet?

A:
Folic acid, the synthetic form of the B vitamin folate, is incredibly important. For one thing, folate is a key regulator of an amino acid called homocysteine, a breakdown product of animal protein. A number of studies have connected high levels of homocysteine in the blood to arterial disease and heart attacks. Folate helps the body eliminate homocysteine from the blood. Recently, Dr. Howard Morrison, an epidemiologist in Ottawa, was able to make a direct connection between folate and heart disease. He looked at folate levels in the blood of 5,056 men who had participated in a nutrition study in the 1970s, and he found that those with low levels of the vitamin were 69 percent more likely to have died from heart problems in the years since.

Folate also has been found to prevent neural tube defects (such as spina bifida and anencephaly) in babies, which are caused when this structure fails to form properly. The neural tube is the embryonic tissue that later becomes the brain and spinal cord. Apparently folic acid is essential to its proper development. Earlier this year, the Food and Drug Administration ordered pasta, rice, and flour makers to add folic acid to their foods as protection against birth defects. This is partly because folic acid plays its important role in neural tube development during the first twenty-eight days of conception—usually before the woman knows she is pregnant—so it doesn't help to tell women to take vitamin supplements during pregnancy.

Folate also may be involved in preventing a whole range of chronic diseases. As the folic acid fortification rule moves into place, we may see a number of health benefits. In fact, since the Morrison study, some doctors are saying the government should double its folic acid RDA (recommended daily allowance), from 200 micrograms to 400 micrograms, to help people protect their hearts.

Folic acid is abundant in dark-green leafy vegetables, carrots, torula yeast, orange juice, asparagus, beans, and wheat germ. But as many as 90 percent of Americans don't get that protective 400 micrograms in their diet—for example, you'd have to eat two cups of steamed spinach, a cup of boiled lentils, or eight oranges every day. So it's important to take a supplement, especially if you're a woman and considering having children someday.

A few cautions, though: Some people are allergic to the folic acid in pills. Also, anyone with a history of convulsive disorder or hormone-related cancer should not take doses above 400 micrograms a day for extended periods. Finally, high levels of folate can mask the signs of vitamin B-12 deficiency. Older people and vegetarians, who are most at risk for deficiencies in B-12, should make sure they're also getting enough of that vitamin if they begin taking folic acid supplements.

How Hazardous Are Food Dyes?

Q:
What's up with Yellow No. 5? I've heard rumors that it contains pig blood, and I am trying to eliminate animal products from my diet.

A:
There is no need for artificial dyes in food. They're put in purely for the convenience of manufacturers. You don't use dyes when you cook at home, so why would you want them in foods you buy? I suggest going through your pantry and throwing out anything that's got artificial color in it. That will be noted on the label as "certified color," "artificial color," or something specific like "FD & C Yellow No. 5" or "Red No. something."

Here's why: Compounds that reflect specific wavelengths of light are energetic molecules that can interact with DNA, potentially causing mutations. Many dyes that were considered safe have since been found to be carcinogenic. They might also weaken our immune systems and speed up aging. Even though artificial dyes have to get approval from the U.S. Food and Drug Administration (and similar agencies in other countries), there's no agreement from country to country as to which ones are safe.

The number you see indicates that the FDA has approved the dye for use in food, drug, and cosmetic products. FD & C Yellow No. 5 is tartrazine, a synthetic dye made from precursor organic compounds with no connection to pig blood. Tartrazine may cause allergies and hyperactivity in children. The FDA has estimated that 50,000 to 100,000 Americans are sensitive to tartrazine and suffer reactions like swelling, asthma, or contact dermatitis. Several hundred products contain the dye, including drugs, cake mixes, lime and lemon beverages, cheese dishes, and fruit-flavored candies. The dye is also used in fabrics.

As a vegetarian, you don't need to worry that food dyes are of animal origin. They are all synthetic chemicals. Their main danger is their carcinogenic potential.

The color of foods contributes to the pleasure of eating. But you don't need artificial colors to enjoy your food. Even though synthetic dyes are so common, I suggest trying hard to avoid them. Natural coloring agents exist and should be used more. Annatto is an orange one made from the seed of a tropical tree and widely used to make margarine yellow and cheese orange. Chlorella is a green pigment derived from algae. Caramel (from burnt sugar) and beet extract are also common. Commercial foods containing them are okay.

Forgetting Something?

Q:

Should I be concerned with forgetting what I was talking about midsentence? It seems like it's getting worse. I'll be saying something and all of a sudden I'll lose my train of thought. Could this be stress? A brain disorder? I am only twenty-seven years old.

A:

Since you're twenty-seven, the cause is probably stress. Stress and anxiety often interfere with memory. Other common causes of memory problems in people in their twenties include smoking marijuana and using other psychoactive drugs like Valium and its relatives, including alcohol.

Memory loss is something to be concerned about. But even with the symptoms you mention, forgetting things is unlikely to be related to a brain disorder in someone your age. I'd like to see what happens if you try some relaxation techniques and eliminate any factors from your life that might be interfering with your memory. The most effective stress reduction technique I know is conscious regulation of breath. For a great breathing exercise see page 233. Regular aerobic exercise and yoga are also good ways to relax and relieve tension.

Another thing to do: Forget about losing your memory. Anxiety about memory can sometimes be a greater problem than actual memory loss, especially in younger people. Americans are particularly susceptible to this. We hear all these public service announcements about Alzheimer's, and they terrify us.

Also, consider how memory works. The secret to memory is attention. If people aren't practiced at paying attention, or don't want to pay attention to what's going on, they aren't going to remember. So the problem may be not memory but attention. And the secret to attention is motivation. Unless you're really motivated to pay attention, you may not remember things. And unless you are really motivated and attentive when communicating with the person you're talking to, you may forget what you're saying.

Is the Fabled G-spot for Real?

Q:
My friend and I have a disagreement over whether a woman's "G" spot is medical fact or psychosomatic fiction. What do you think?

A:
The G-spot has not been accepted as medical fact, although many sexologists believe that it may bring about vaginal orgasm. Still, many men and women say they have located it. I even know of one feminist writer who was politically opposed to the idea of a G-spot, but who now says it's real after taking a workshop in tantric sex.

The G-spot is named after a man named Grafenberg, who first described it. If you want to experiment with finding it, the best method is for the woman to sit atop the man, facing his feet. Then you can experiment with finding the spot, which is inside the vagina between the cervix and the pubic bone. If you're flying solo, you can search for it yourself.

Another way is to study tantra, the ancient Indian art of using sexual energy to connect with the divine intimacy. Tantra workshops are now being offered around the country, but as it's being taught today, this tantra might not have any relationship to Indian tantra. One of the main techniques being taught, however, is finding the G-spot and massaging it. Proponents of modern tantra claim that women experience incredible orgasms because of this stimulation and ejaculate large volumes of fluid. The idea isn't new: ancient Chinese sexual philosophy called female ejaculation "the tide of Yin."

I wouldn't get too obsessed with finding a magical spot as the center for female pleasure. Anxiety and emphasis on orgasm can be the quickest route to unhappy sexual experience. Have fun exploring, and stay in touch with the intimacy and pleasure of lovemaking.

Ginger as an Anti-Inflammatory?

Q:

You recommended ginger to cure wrist tendinitis. I have some tendinitis in both of my wrists and also am beginning to have pains in my lower thumb joints. I have been consuming large amounts of cooked ginger in a fried form. Is this the amount that should make a detectable difference? (I am talking about thin slices of a knob or two of a piece of ginger.)

A:

You may not be getting enough of ginger's anti-inflammatory effect with the cooked fresh ginger. The preferred form for this use is the powder. My preference would be to start with one capsule of 500 milligrams of ginger twice a day with food. You can go up to two capsules twice a day with food. You can also use as much fresh ginger as you like in preparing your food. But keep in mind that fresh ginger is not as rich in anti-inflammatory components as dried ginger.

Ginger's effect on inflammation is documented in several studies. A possible mechanism of action involves a change in the synthesis of prostaglandins and leucotrienes—hormones that mediate inflammation.

Ginger is usually called a root, but it's actually a rhizome, an underground stem of a tropical plant, *Zingiber officinale*. Besides having anti-inflammatory propperties, ginger works well as a treatment for nausea and motion sickness—probably the use for which it is most valued. Its efficiency is attributed to the volatile oil that gives ginger its characteristic pungency. Ginger also tones the cardiovascular system and reduces platelet aggregation, helping to protect against heart attacks and strokes.

How Dangerous Are Hair Dyes?

Q:
Is it safe to use hair dyes regularly?

A:
In general, I discourage people from using hair dyes. Artificial colors are suspect in cosmetic products, just as they are in food. When you apply hair dyes to your head, they are absorbed through the scalp into the many blood vessels that supply it. There is suspicion that hair dyes can increase risk of bladder cancer, because when they are absorbed, they concentrate in the bladder. Dark dyes are of particular concern, because they contain more chemicals than light ones.

I was surprised to learn that about half of all women in the United States dye their hair—an increase of about 50 percent in the past decade. And the hair-dye market for middle-aged men is expected to grow rapidly—already one in eight men between the ages of thirteen and seventy uses dyes. Commercial hair-dye makers sell $7 billion worth of their products worldwide every year.

The most recent research on hair dyes and cancer, a seven-year study of 573,369 women by the American Cancer Society, didn't find a significantly increased risk. Women who used very dark dyes over a period of twenty years or more did show a greater tendency to develop bone cancer and non-Hodgkin's lymphoma, however. It has been suggested that dyes could have been a cause of Jacqueline Onassis's cancer. And other studies *have* associated an increased risk of cancer with hair dyes.

Cancer or no, dyes aren't very healthy for your hair. They can cause it to become brittle and to break easily. Curiously, hair dyes aren't subject to Food and Drug Administration requirements for safety testing; they were exempted in 1938.

I would stay away from chemical dyes. If you use them, make sure you don't leave them on your head any longer than necessary. Rinse your scalp thoroughly with water when you're done. Wear gloves during the whole process.

Henna, a plant-derived dye, is okay to use. And you can find other natural dyes in health food stores. I would stick with those.

Help for Halitosis?

Q:
*I'm concerned about the causes of and natural reme-
dies for bad breath.*

A:
The usual cause of bad breath is bacteria growing
on the tongue, and sometimes around the gum line,
too. There are a couple of simple ways to take care
of the problem. First, try a tongue scraper. This is a
metal instrument that you use to scrape your tongue
once or twice a day, cleaning off bacteria. Second, you
can brush your tongue with a germicidal toothpaste
when you're brushing your teeth. Just take an extra
thirty seconds to brush your tongue after you're done
with your teeth, and try to include the back of your
tongue—which will take some practice.

One product that works well is chlorine dioxide,
which is in some regular toothpastes (for instance,
Oxyfresh). Or go to a health food store and look for a
toothpaste containing tea tree oil, an extract from the
leaves of *Melaleuca alternifolia,* an Australian tree.
Tea tree oil is a safe, powerful disinfectant that smells
a bit like eucalyptus.

For temporary breath problems—say, when you return to work after a garlic-and-onion-laden lunch—try
chewing on a bit of parsley or some fennel seeds.
These will freshen your breath and also offer a nice

finish to a meal. Try to stay away from products like Certs and BreathSavers; they contain aspartame.

Bad breath is sometimes associated with gum disease. Check your gums for signs of irritation or swelling. If you notice a problem, talk to your dentist about it (he or she may refer you to a periodontist). Constant bad breath also may be a sign of systemic illness, especially liver disease or kidney disease. If it's a systemic problem, the breath is likely to have a distinct smell. Liver problems produce a mousy odor; severe bronchial infections will smell rotten. Sinusitis and inflammation inside the nose can also cause bad breath.

I wouldn't pay much attention to the claims made about mouthwashes like Scope or Listerine. These germicidal formulas may help, but they often don't penetrate into the crevices of the tongue. That's why I prefer brushing the tongue.

Cure for Hangovers?

Q:

I hate getting out of bed to find myself with quite a splitting reminder of the night before. Is there anything that can help cure the common hangover?

A:

Alcohol is a strong toxin to both the liver and the nervous system, and it irritates the upper digestive tract and urinary system as well. The morning after a binge, you also feel the effects of dehydration. Everyone has a cure for a hangover: sailors claim salt water is the antidote; the Egyptians ate boiled cabbage as a preventive; today, many folks claim it's the "hair of the dog" that'll stop the hammering. Believe what you will.

I probably don't need to say that moderation is the best way to avoid hangovers. It makes sense to imbibe as much water as possible while you're drinking alcohol, to avoid dehydration. Taking aspirin before drinking, though popular, doesn't help. The best and only surefire remedy is time: as your body metabolizes the toxic overdose, symptoms subside. If you have access to pure oxygen in a canister you can try inhaling some to see if it speeds recovery, but I doubt this is practical for most people. I recommend taking a B-complex vitamin supplement plus extra thiamine (100 milligrams) to counter the B-vitamin depletion caused by alcohol, along with several doses of milk thistle (*Silybum marianum*) to protect the liver. But I really don't know of any hangover treatment that works as well as putting time between yourself and the night before.

Be aware that you should pick your poison wisely. Since alcohol is exempt from most labeling requirements, it may contain additives that can trigger asthma, migraines, and other reactions. Whenever possible, choose quality brands. The extra money you pour out for a premium cocktail may tax your wallet but will help your liver love you.

Some distilled beverages are rich in substances called congeners, toxic impurities that can greatly add to your woes. Bourbon, rum, and cognac are particularly "dirty." Champagne and some sweet wines are also notorious causers of hangovers. Vodka, being just pure alcohol and water, is the cleanest.

It's always a good idea to pace yourself, and to eat if you have more than a drink or two.

My drink of choice is sake, which seems pretty clean to me. I don't get a hangover from it, even when I drink more than normal. *Kanpai!*

Natural Remedies for Hay Fever?

Q:
During the spring and summer I suffer from minor hay fever (sneezing, irritated and swollen sinuses). For years I've kept it under control with over-the-counter drugs like Sudafed. I'd like to stop taking these drugs. Are there any natural remedies?

A:
As you've found, conventional treatments for hay fever aren't very good. Desensitization shots are expensive, can hurt, and are risky. Antihistamines often reduce itching, dry up a runny nose, and quiet down a sneezing attack, but because they act on the brain, they can make you drowsy and depressed. Recently, new antihistamines have been developed that aren't absorbed into the brain (Claritin, for example). They may have different side effects, they don't work for everyone, and they're not cheap. Steroid drugs are even stronger than antihistamines. Doctors often prescribe steroid nasal inhalers (like Beconase and Vancenase) for hay fever. They can be very effective, but the steroids are bound to get into your system, and these hormones weaken our immune systems.

My objection to all these drugs is that they suppress or block the allergic process and, in doing so, only perpetuate the disease by frustrating it. I've had intense ragweed allergy all my life and I know that it's possible to make things better by changing your lifestyle and attitude.

Stinging nettle (*Urtica dioica*) is the best natural remedy that I know. It's most effective taken in a freeze-dried form sold as a capsule. This product is available from the Eclectic Institute (see Other Resources, page 292). The dose is one to two capsules every two to four hours as needed. Stinging nettle is completely nontoxic and spectacularly effective in controlling hay fever symptoms.

What to Do for Cracked, Dry Heels?

Q:
I have dry, cracked skin on my heels. I eat a healthy vegetarian diet and I scrub my heels with pumice to exfoliate the dead skin. Are the cracks a symptom of something else? Can you suggest a remedy?

A:
Problem dry heels are just that: dry heels. They're a common occurrence, especially in dry climates, and may show up seasonally. I have a big problem with them here in the desert because the heel cracks can become very painful if dirt gets in them or if they become deep.

Typically, if you wear socks, you'll regain the moisture on your heels and the cracks will go away. But I like to go barefoot or wear sandals. So it's an ongoing battle.

The key consideration for problem dry heels is finding a way to keep the cracks clean. The first thing I've found that really works to repair them is instant acrylic glue. It may sound crazy, but you just put a drop or two in the cleaned crack and press the edges together. The glue seals the skin and allows the healing to take place very quickly, often overnight. This also works for cracked fingertips.

Another possibility is to go to a pedicurist and get some professional loving-kindness directed at your feet. You can get footbaths, have the dead skin scraped off, and even get your toenails painted, if you like that kind of thing.

You may also want to try adding as much moisture as you can to your heels and feet. Water alone will extract moisture when it evaporates from your skin; oil protects, but can't add moisture. So the best moisturizer combines both.

Anything that stimulates circulation is also helpful: for example, a steam sauna with a cool water rinse between spells of heat.

Help for Hemorrhoids?

Q:

Being one of the masses who have desk jobs and take numerous plane trips, I often have hemorrhoids. Can you suggest any alternatives to the standard over-the-counter remedies?

A:

Hemorrhoids are distended veins around the anus that can become inflamed, causing itching, pain, and bleeding. They're not unusual at all; in fact, most people are bothered by them at some time or other. The pain can become severe. Prolonged sitting, constipation, and irritants in the diet are common causes. So is pregnancy. Stress can also make hemorrhoids flare up. Dietary irritants include strong spices such as red pepper and mustard, and drinks such as coffee, decaffeinated coffee, and alcohol. Avoid these, and tobacco.

You can treat constipation by eating more fiber. A vegetarian diet will help you here. Or take psyllium seed husks, in any of the forms available in drugstores and health food stores. Triphala, an herbal mixture from the Ayurvedic tradition, is an excellent bowel regulator. You can buy it in capsules in health food stores. Follow the dosage on the label. Drink lots of water—more than you think you need.

A natural, soothing treatment for the hemorrhoids

themselves is an old-fashioned sitz bath. Sit in a bath-tub filled with enough warm water to cover the anal area for fifteen minutes several times a day. Also, apply aloe vera gel to the area frequently. Instead of dry toilet paper, which will irritate the veins, use compresses of witch hazel to clean the anal area after bowel movements. You can buy witch hazel at any drugstore. Just moisten sheets of toilet paper with it. There are also pre-moistened, pre-packaged versions available.

Finally, here are two Chinese remedies that use foods to correct the imbalances that may cause hemorrhoids: Eat an orange three times a day, or eat two bananas first thing in the morning.

Why the Wait for Herbal Benefits?

Q:

In many of your discussions about vitamins and herbs, you say it may take up to two months before you see results. Why does it take so long before we can notice any benefits?

A:

As a society we're used to taking purified drugs, powerful agents that typically produce immediate effects. When you're using herbal treatments, you're working with dilute, much weaker preparations. Natural remedies require you to think about health and medicine in a different way. We've become conditioned by pharmaceuticals to expect quick, dramatic responses in our bodies. But often, these drugs are only suppressing symptoms, rather than treating the root problem. With natural medicine, you're reaching more deeply into the body's systems to create lasting health.

Herbs often contain families of active ingredients, instead of one concentrated, powerhouse chemical. They may include elements that soften the impact of the main component, or that create other effects. There are important differences between taking a caffeine tablet and drinking a cup of coffee. Or snorting cocaine instead of chewing on a coca leaf.

Often when you use herbs and vitamins as remedies, you're working to change body chemistry and physiology, rather than simply suppress symptoms. In order to see the more profound changes, a certain amount of time is required. And often the changes will be subtle.

Some herbal treatments and other natural remedies can work quickly. One example is stinging nettle (*Urtica dioica*) for hay fever. It relieves symptoms rapidly and without toxicity, with the added bonus of providing trace minerals. Other speedy solutions include the ancient medicinal plant ephedra (*Ephedra sinica*) for acute asthma attacks, and licorice extract (not red licorice twists!) for stomach distress. And when you get a cold or the flu, you can expect echinacea, the purple coneflower (*Echinacea purpurea*) to help out quickly. But in many cases, such as when using Saint-John's-wort (*Hypericum perforatum*) to treat depression, it can take six to eight weeks before you notice changes. It may also take that long for you to be reasonably sure it's the herb making the difference, not a visit from a friend or a pleasant surprise at work. With any of these herbs, you may see results sooner, but my point is to be patient when you're using natural remedies.

Can I Take an Herbal Overdose?

Q:

I would like to know whether there is any herb that one could consume to excess and therefore suffer health problems. I consume 25 grams of raw ginger, 25 grams of raw garlic, and 20 grams of eleuthero (Siberian ginseng) every day. Are there any dangers in doing so? I also plan to take triphala, ashwagandha, barley green, sun chlorella, echinacea, Gingko biloba, and gotu kola. Is there any harm in taking any of these products in the same or larger quantities?

A:

That's a lot of herbs to take every day, and I have to wonder what health problems you're using them for. In general, I think it's a shame to waste medicinal herbs by taking them just because they're there. They'll work better for you if you save them for the times when your body needs special attention.

I think any herb can be taken in excess. For example, there have been a few reported cases of bleeding problems in people taking very large amounts of garlic, which can act as an anticoagulant. Some herbalists also say that too much garlic can deplete your intestinal flora and make it harder to absorb nutrients.

I think the amounts of ginger and garlic you're talking about are fine. But I wonder about swallowing a whole grab bag of herbs, unless you're taking them for specific reasons.

Herbs are dilute forms of natural drugs, not health foods or dietary supplements. You shouldn't take them casually or for no reason, any more than you would take pharmaceutical drugs casually or for no reason. Any herb that produces a therapeutic effect can also cause side effects. And, just as for any drug, it's important to watch for sensitivities particular to your body.

Unless you have specific illnesses you are treating, I'd back off from the herbal cornucopia. If you use herbs just because you think it's healthy to do so, you may build up a resistance to their effects. Then you won't have them available to work for you if you get sick and really need them.

Healing Remedies for Herpes?

Q:

What do you recommend for treating genital herpes? I've tried acyclovir, and I've found it interrupts the virus's behavior but does nothing for healing the body. I've also been taking L-lysine three times a day and have found this to be effective. While I'm at it: Any thoughts about treating herpes on the lips?

A:

As you learned, acyclovir is less than ideal. It's expensive, may have side effects, and merely suppresses the symptoms without correcting the problem. L-lysine, an amino acid present in various foods, is worth trying because it inhibits replication of the herpes virus. I recommend 500 to 1,000 milligrams a day on an empty stomach. You can enhance L-lysine's effectiveness by minimizing foods like nuts, seeds, peas, and chocolate. In my experience, L-lysine is more effective with oral herpes than genital.

You might want to experiment with another natural product: red marine algae (of the family *Dumontiaceae*), marketed under the name Intracept Pro (made by In Life Energy Systems). In lab tests, red marine algae appears to inhibit the herpes virus, although definitive human tests are lacking.

Many people have seen their herpes go into complete remission as a result of changes in lifestyle and mental attitude. Others have experienced significantly fewer flare-ups after trying visualizations and mental affirmations that tell the virus it's welcome in the body as long as it stays in the dormant stage. There's definitely the possibility of living in balance with the organism even if you can't get rid of it.

Got the Hiccups?

Q:
How best to get rid of hiccups?

A:
Hiccups are spasms of the diaphragm, followed by sudden closure of the glottis (the opening between the vocal cords), which temporarily stops the inflow of air. They can result from stress, excitement, stomach irritation, toxins, temperature changes, and other triggers. The root cause is irritability of the phrenic nerves along the spinal column; these nerves control the diaphragm.

Sometimes hiccups go away within a few minutes, and sometimes they last a long time. The longest-term sufferer known was an American pig farmer who hiccuped from 1922 to 1987.

Hiccups often resist the most ingenious treatment methods, so it's good to have several options in mind. You can try standing on your head, or swallowing crushed ice or dry bread, or drinking a glass of water rapidly. Another remedy is to make ginger tea and add honey, then sip it for ten minutes. Some people swear by putting a teaspoon of sugar or honey on the back of the tongue and swallowing it slowly. One remedy I've never had a chance to try involves drinking from a glass of water with a spoon in it while touching the end of the spoon to one ear. Another is asking a good friend to shout "boo" unexpectedly and scare you into breathing evenly.

My favorite method is to breathe in and out of a paper bag held over the nose and the mouth. This raises the carbon dioxide level of the blood, calming the phrenic nerves and diaphragm. (Don't use a plastic bag, though, because it can cling to your nostrils.) Keep breathing into the paper bag until the hiccups stop, or you feel uncomfortable.

Need a Quickie for a Hickey?

Q:
What's the best way to get rid of a hickey?

A:
First of all, there's no quick fix for a hickey. It's just a plain old bruise, and basically you wait for it to heal. My advice is to tell your partner either not to kiss so hard next time or not to kiss so high above your collar line. You could try ice right away on the injured area, but that might interrupt the heat of the moment. (A friend of mine puts a tablespoon in his freezer and then applies the cold spoon to the hickey for the same effect.) Fortunately, hickeys aren't life-threatening or permanently disfiguring; like any bruise, they'll begin to fade in a few days. If you're shy about walking around with a red splotch on your neck, try my favorite remedy: a turtleneck.

You can experiment with a few things while you wait it out. Rub in a little tincture of arnica or arnica gel. Arnica comes from a plant in the daisy family that grows in the Rocky Mountains, and it's wonderful for bruises, sprains, and sore muscles. Aloe vera, from a succulent plant native to Africa, also soothes skin irritation. Kathi Keville, author of *Herbs for Health and Healing,* makes a bruise compress with the following:

1 tablespoon tincture of arnica
a smidgen of Saint-John's-wort flowering tops
a smidgen of witch hazel bark or chamomile flowers
4 drops lavender essential oil
2 tablespoons cold water

Soak a washcloth in the liquid, wring it out, and place it directly on your hickey.

Home Tests for HIV?

Q:

Are over-the-counter HIV tests accurate or reliable?

A:

The Food and Drug Administration approved home HIV tests after a great deal of debate. When the first tests were submitted for regulatory scrutiny, there was much concern about accuracy. On top of that, the FDA and some AIDS activists worried that people would not get the psychological help they needed when they learned the results of positive tests. This information can be extremely upsetting. People who are tested at clinics or by their doctors always receive their results in person—from a trained professional. Counseling is critical to understanding what the results mean, learning how to cope with them, and finding out about treatment (if one is infected). Many people feel there is just no substitute for face-to-face counseling.

The FDA ultimately decided that the tests were highly accurate and that they assured patient anonymity and provided appropriate counseling. It was thought that this option would allow more people to be tested and to know their HIV status, which in turn could stem the tide of new infections. In one survey, many people said they preferred the home test to going to a clinic. Men of color in particular said they were more likely to use a home test kit. And according to the Centers for Disease Control and Prevention, 85 percent of people tested in clinics don't get counseling with the results.

If it's more convenient and you decide you don't want to talk to someone in person, I think a home test is fine. Just make sure you do make use of the counseling available by phone.

The Confide HIV testing service, from a subsidiary of Johnson & Johnson, put out the first home kit on the market. In data submitted to regulators, the kit was 99.95 percent accurate in identifying 3,940 samples of uninfected blood. It also correctly picked out all of the 150 samples infected with HIV, the virus that causes AIDS. In mid-1997, Johnson & Johnson pulled the Confide test from the market, claiming that only 90,000 tests had been processed during the previous year and that demand wasn't expected to grow. The FDA had also sent two warning letters to the company regarding the test, so it's not entirely clear why the product was pulled.

The standard Home Access test costs $29.95 for results by phone within seven days. The "express" Home Access test is $49.95 for results within three days. Call 800 HIV TEST (448-8378) for more information.

Here's how the test works: You start by reading the instructions and pretest counseling booklet, which are in both Spanish and English. Then you prick your finger with a fingerstick in the kit and collect a blood sample. You drip three drops of blood onto a test card marked with a special identification number, and you mail it to a laboratory for HIV-antibody testing. Seven days later, you call a toll-free number, day or night, for the results. If the results are negative, an auto- mated voice tells you so. If they are positive, you talk to a live person about them, what they mean, and how to get medical care.

It's very important to stay on the phone and talk to the counselor once you get the result. Realize that false positives do occur, so if you test positive, you should get tested again. The lab will do a second test by the same method, and if that one's positive, will perform a more sophisticated test called the Western blot.

If you test positive, the counselor will tell you about a number of drugs that lengthen life expectancy. You can also find out about medical, psychological, and legal services available to you.

Also, keep in mind that a negative result doesn't mean you never have to worry about HIV again. If you're sexually active in a nonmonogamous situation, or if you inject drugs, it's important to get tested regularly. There is a "window" period of up to six months where you may be infected without the virus's showing up on a test.

And always use a condom or a dental dam to protect yourself during sexual intercourse. If you do inject drugs, use a clean needle.

Kombucha Tea for HIV?

Q:
I'm infected with HIV and am wondering what you think about the Kombucha mushroom for someone with a weakened immune system. I've been drinking the tea for two months and so far consider the effects nothing short of miraculous.

A:
First, the Kombucha mushroom is not a mushroom. It's a mixed culture of several species of bacteria and yeasts that is reported to have immune-boosting and antibiotic properties. Kombucha has become popular because of some initial positive press about its beneficial effects and because it's readily available.

If you're getting good effects, go ahead and use it. But generally I'm cautious about recommending it for two reasons. The first is that the culture can become contaminated with dangerous organisms; this would be of special concern for anyone whose immune system was suppressed. There are reports of a number of serious reactions, including deaths, among users of Kombucha mushrooms apparently due to contamination. If the culture develops an unusual odor or color, throw it out. Second, I'm not enthusiastic about people taking antibiotics of any kind without good reason.

I've heard a few dramatic stories of improvement among people with HIV and reports of higher energy

levels and mental acuity. But we really have no research on Kombucha. All of the reports, like yours, are
testimonials. People with HIV who have low T-cell
counts should be sure to talk to their physician before
taking Kombucha.

In general the people with HIV who have done well
are those who are using the protease "cocktail" (a
powerful combination of anti-HIV drugs) and who
have worked to improve their total lifestyle—diet,
stress reduction, exercise, sexuality, and emotional
life.

What's the Buzz on Hives?

Q:
I get hives when my body temperature rises. What is the cause of this? I break out in a rash and experience profound itching. Please help me!

A:
You have an instability of the histamine system. Histamine is a biological response modifier, which is released in inflammatory and allergic reactions. Hives are very common, with about 20 percent of people experiencing them at one time or another. You're a long way toward a solution by noticing what triggers the itchy, rash-like bumps. In some people, hives can be set off by stress; in others, by food sensitivities, and in still others by the kind of temperature changes you describe. Three-quarters of the time, the reaction disappears within about eight months. It almost always goes away within a couple of years.

Conventional medicine is not of great help here. I would recommend that you try a course of quercetin. Quercetin is a bioflavonoid from buckwheat and citrus fruits. It works by stabilizing the membranes of cells that release histamine, bringing allergic reactions under control. You can buy quercetin products in health food stores. The best form is a coated 400-milligram tablet, taken twice a day between meals.

Cornstarch or colloidal oatmeal added to your bathwater can soothe the itching. Aveeno bath treatment, available at drugstores, is one good oatmeal product.

You may also want to include plenty of garlic and onions in your diet, since they decrease histamine production.

Keep in mind that emotional upsets and stress are a very important trigger of hives: there is a definite mind-body connection with the histamine system. I would recommend working with a hypnotherapist or practitioner of visualization therapy who can help you quiet the condition.

Holistic Medicine for the People?

Q:
Natural medicine has become the upper-middle-class rage. Dr. Deepak Chopra charges thousands of dollars for his seminars. We have a doctor here in Maine who is a famous holistic practitioner for women, but won't take Medicaid patients. It costs $1,000 to be taught transcendental meditation. How and when are we going to provide alternative medicine to the poor?

A:
That's a very good question. You're quite correct that alternative medicine is available mostly to the affluent, and until insurance companies see the wisdom of paying practitioners, I think it will be hard to change the situation.

Be aware, however, that doctors like myself always try to provide patients with information about managing common ailments on their own with therapies that are cost-effective and easily available. Many elements of natural medicine are not expensive. Breathing exercises, dietary adjustment, and the use of herbs are all low-cost ways to better health. Even special treatments like acupuncture may cost much less than mainstream ones.

Some insurance companies are realizing they can save money by offering to pay for alternative care. And some groups of patients and health practitioners are lobbying for better coverage. A 1993 Harvard Medical School report found that Americans were making almost as many visits to alternative caregivers as to conventional physicians. A study by the American Western Life Insurance Company that compared conventional treatment to alternative care demonstrated some striking cost savings.

American Western Life, in Foster City, California, maintains a special plan that covers alternative care by naturopaths and specialists including acupuncturists, hypnotherapists, reflexologists, and experts in herbal medicine. It has a twenty-four-hour advice hotline for herbal remedies. Alternative Health Insurance Services, a health maintenance organization in Thousand Oaks, California, also covers a range of approaches, from Ayurvedic to traditional Chinese medicine. Blue Cross of Washington & Alaska, based in Mountlake Terrace, Washington, is creating an alternative medicine benefit plan, as is Oxford Health Plans in the Northeast. In the state of Washington, health plans are required by law to provide access to licensed chiropractors, acupuncturists, and naturopaths. Shop around: you may find insurance companies that are starting to include natural medicine in their plans.

Help for Hot Flashes?

Q:
I have tried herb after herb and I still can't find the right combination to get rid of my hot flashes. I'm desperate. Can you help?

A:
It's interesting how medicine has transformed a natural phase in the cycle of women's bodies into a disorder. For many years, it was considered impolite to even mention the word (that's when menopause was referred to as "the change"). Then menopause became one in a long list of imbalances attributed to women's reproductive systems, with proper intervention mandated. Pharmaceutical companies and gynecologists bombard women with the same message: Menopause is a time of unhappiness, bringing moodiness, hot flashes, osteoporosis, and loss of youthful attractiveness. The "life change" is actually a deficiency disease, the theory goes, and so only estrogen replacement therapy can restore vibrancy to women's bodies.

I'd recommend looking at this time of life in a new way. Instead of signifying aging and the loss of childbearing ability, menopause can be a time to discover new energy, a freer self, and deeper wisdom within. Yes, there are discomforts associated with the changes in your body during this time. But these are signs of an opportunity to discover and claim the power of the second half of life.

During menopause, your body is adjusting to a change in hormone production. The ovaries stop releasing eggs, and it's no longer possible to get pregnant. The pituitary hormones, follicle-stimulating hormone (FSH), and luteinizing hormone (LH), which normally cycle during the month, begin to flow continuously at high levels. The ovaries slow down their output of estrogen, progesterone, and androgens. At the same time, other sites, such as the adrenal gland, the skin, and the brain, may take over hormone production. The ease of the transition depends greatly on a woman's stress level, emotional health, and nutritional status.

We rarely hear about women who have few problems with menopause, even though there are many of them. In non-Western cultures, menopause is often considered a time of strengthening and health for women. So first of all, it's important not to buy into the negative images and attitudes surrounding menopause in our culture.

Around 85 percent of American women experience the hot flashes you mention during menopause. Not long ago, Jane Fonda described her first hot flash this way: "When Ted and I were courting at a sound-and-light show in Athens, Greece, I had my first hot flash. It was dramatic and kind of exciting." You may feel a great heat around your head and neck, sweat profusely, then feel chilled. Some women go through these episodes for a few months, some for years. Hot flashes have been linked to blocked energy and unused sexual potential, so women who fear they will lose their sex drive with menopause may be more bothered by them. One tactic is to work to free your sexual energy and overcome the messages you are getting about an expected loss of sex drive.

I personally recommend a menopausal formula that works well for most women. Buy capsules or tinctures of these herbs at a health food store: dong quai, a female tonic made from the root of *Angelica sinensis;* vitex, or chaste tree (*Vitex agnus-castus*), a regulator of the female reproductive system; and damiana (*Turnera diffusa*), a plant that has a reputation as a tonic and female aphrodisiac. Take two capsules of each of these every day at noon, or one dropperful of each tincture mixed in warm water once a day at noon. Keep taking the herbs until you don't experience any hot flashes, then begin to reduce the dose and try to stop altogether.

Another herb widely used for menopausal discomforts, including hot flashes, is black cohosh (*Cimifuga racemosa*), now available in a commercial product called Remifemin. Its effectiveness is supported by good scientific data.

Many women also find ginseng to be very helpful for hot flashes, especially in combination with vitamin E (800 IU a day of the natural form). Nutrition is also important. Soy products contain estrogenlike substances that may account for the low incidence of menopausal symptoms in Japanese women. And researchers have found that deep, slow breathing can reduce hot flashes by half, probably by calming the central nervous system.

Finally, there are other Chinese herbs that help to relieve the problem. I'd suggest you visit a practitioner of traditional Chinese medicine if you want to learn about them.

How to Get Unleaded?

Q:

My son has lead poisoning. What will the treatment be?

A:

Lead poisoning of fetuses and young children is a serious problem in the United States. Even low-level lead exposure can cause hyperactivity, learning disabilities, and growth problems over time. High levels of lead can reduce intelligence, cause severe retardation, and even lead to early death. It's very important to test for lead in young children because they are so susceptible to its effects, particularly as their brains develop. Plus, there is so much lead in the environment that it is easy for them to get exposed. If your drinking water contains more than 10 parts per billion of lead, you and your family can consume enough of this heavy metal to cause problems.

The most common sources of lead are water from lead pipes, flakes of lead paint in older homes, lead glazes on pottery, and lead from older processing equipment and fuels that ends up in canned vegetables. Get rid of all known sources of lead. You should find out what your pipes are made of and get your water tested for lead content. Or you can purchase a home purifying system (see page 273) that will remove lead and other heavy metals. The Centers for

Disease Control and Prevention suggests that every child under age six be tested for lead poisoning.

I recommend two precautions to reduce the chance of ingesting lead from household water. First, let the water run from the tap for three to five minutes after any period of nonuse. Second, don't draw water from the hot tap—even for cooking—because hot water leaches out impurities much more readily than cold, and because it is likely to have picked up impurities from the hot-water tank. (No matter what your pipes are made of, water from the hot tap is unfit for human consumption.)

If you detect lead poisoning early, there are effective ways to treat it. The American Association of Naturopathic Physicians recommends a nutritional approach. The antioxidants—vitamins A, C, and E, plus selenium—can help detoxify the body and protect nerve tissue from damage. Zinc and vitamin C help reduce harm from the lead, and vitamin A may counter infections that lead-poisoned children tend to suffer. The association also suggests a regimen of herbs and amino acids to detoxify the liver.

If lead poisoning is confirmed, I would be inclined to go for conventional treatment: chelation therapy. Injected or oral chelating agents bond with lead, allowing the child to excrete the metal in the urine. The newest oral medicine is Succimer, or DMSA. The treatment normally lasts nineteen days and should go no longer than three weeks. Side effects of chelation therapy can include rash, nausea, and a loss of appetite, but the benefits of getting the lead out are much greater than the risks of therapy.

Better Methods for Treating Lupus?

Q:

Are there any homeopathic medicines that are good for treating lupus?

A:

Lupus is a serious autoimmune disease that is imperfectly managed by conventional medicine. It can be mild or life-threatening and may cause a variety of symptoms, including arthritis, skin eruptions, neurological problems, and kidney disease. Four times as many women as men have lupus, and there isn't much known about its cause. Some think a viral infection may trigger the immune-system dysfunction.

The drugs that conventional doctors use for lupus are immune-suppressive and toxic. They may be necessary when symptoms are most severe, but they reduce the chance that the disease will go into remission naturally.

Homeopathic medicine would not be my first choice to treat lupus. Instead, I've seen very good results in patients who modify their diet and use anti-inflammatory supplements and herbs like black currant oil, ginger, turmeric, and feverfew, in addition to mind-body healing techniques like hypnotherapy and guided imagery.

You may also want to experiment with Native American, Ayurvedic, or Chinese medicine. I'd start by eating as little protein as possible and eliminating dairy. Try to get lots of starches and fresh fruits and vegetables.

Eat sardines packed in sardine oil (without salt) three times a week, or take supplemental flaxseed meal. These provide omega-3 fatty acids. Black currant oil is a natural source of another fatty acid called gamma linolenic acid (GLA), which is an effective anti-inflammatory. Take 500 milligrams twice a day. Take feverfew (*Tanacetum parthenium*), an anti-inflammatory herb, to help with any arthritis (one capsule of the freeze-dried leaves twice a day for as long as you notice symptoms).

Exercise regularly. If you're hurting from arthritis, swimming can bring relief. Drink plenty of water and get lots of rest. Seek out ways to avoid stress and fatigue in your life.

It's especially important not to stay with a conventional doctor who encourages you to feel hopeless or negative. Lupus has a high potential to go naturally into remission, and the attitude of your physician can powerfully influence your ability to feel well. For insight into one woman's encounters with conventional and alternative medicine in her efforts to manage this disease, read Laura Chester's book *Lupus Novice: Towards Self-Healing*.

How to Lick Lyme Disease?

Q:
We live in a wooded area in central Wisconsin and often have deer in our backyard. What is a safe way to protect our two-year-old son and ourselves from ticks? Are products like Deep Woods Off! safe for small children? Our son has already had two ticks on him this year. (I don't think they were deer ticks as they were pretty large.) Any info on ticks and Lyme disease would be appreciated.

A:
Lyme disease is an infection caused by an organism called *Borrelia burgdorferi*. It's named after Old Lyme, Connecticut, where doctors discovered the disease when they thought they were dealing with an epidemic of juvenile rheumatoid arthritis. There were about 8,000 cases of it in the United States in 1993, the most recent year for which I have figures.

Lyme disease presents a curious situation. There's a tremendous fascination with it as an exotic illness. And people are fearful of it because the symptoms can persist years after infection, even with treatment. So there's a tendency to rush to this diagnosis whenever patients have strange, persistent symptoms.

At the same time, a definitive diagnosis is often missed. Some physicians don't think to look for it and thus fail to give the proper treatment. To further complicate matters, we don't have a conclusive test for Lyme disease and there's no way of being sure it is the cause of any specific symptom.

Lyme disease is usually treated with up to one month of antibiotics. If these are administered at the right time in the right way, they should eradicate the organism.

If the disease is left untreated, about two-thirds of people infected develop recurring bouts of arthritis—sometimes years after the initial infection. The disease has also been associated with neurological symptoms, although it's not clear how severe they may be.

As you say, deer ticks host the organism. Deer, deer mice, and field mice carry the ticks, which are so small, they're practically invisible until fully engorged with blood—and then they are still hard to see. So the ticks you saw were not deer ticks. You should find out whether deer ticks are present in your area, and if so, whether they carry the bacteria that causes Lyme disease.

Generally I don't recommend any chemical pesticides. The only safe insecticide is pyrethrin, which is made from the flowers of certain chrysanthemum relatives. In areas where the disease is really prevalent, like Long Island and Connecticut, the best prevention is to wear protective clothing when you go out into the woods. Wear light colors and long sleeves, and tuck your pants into your socks. When you get back, wash immediately and keep an eye out for anything unusual on your body.

If you do have any odd symptoms like strange skin rashes, fever, or joint pain, go to a doctor who is knowledgeable about diagnosing and treating Lyme disease. The typical presentation is a rash in concentric rings, like a bull's-eye. But in many cases the rash is not present.

How Bad
Is MSG?

Q:
How can MSG affect me?

A:
People react variably to monosodium glutamate, or MSG. Some people seem to be very sensitive to it, responding with nasal congestion, itching, flushing, headache, chest pain, and nausea. In its full-blown form, this reaction has been called "MSG symptom complex" by the medical establishment and "Chinese restaurant syndrome" by others.

MSG is found in many processed foods and ethnic cuisines. Chinese restaurants often add large amounts of it to stir-fried dishes. It's also used as a flavor enhancer in Japanese cooking, and it is common in packaged soups and sauces. The exact flavor MSG confers is difficult to describe; many just say it increases the "taste intensity" of food. One thing is certain: it makes people thirsty, encouraging them to eat and drink more. Americans consume about 28,000 tons of MSG per year, according to one estimate, reported in the *Journal of Environmental Health* (June 1995).

Chemically, MSG is one type of glutamate, a family of substances derived from glutamic acid, which in turn is one of the building blocks of proteins. "Free glutamate" like MSG is released by the breakdown of protein molecules. Some foods, including fresh tomatoes, tomato paste, and Parmesan cheese, naturally contain free glutamates. Monosodium glutamate was discovered in 1908 by Japanese researcher Kikunae Ikeda, who was looking for the flavor Japanese cooks prize in sea tangles, a type of sea vegetable. Scientists later learned to synthesize MSG as a pure crystalline substance.

Some doctors still dispute the existence of MSG symptom complex, while others believe it's an inherited allergic reaction. People who crusade against MSG cite a series of animal studies, using large amounts of MSG administered orally and by injection to rats and mice, that found the flavoring agent caused lesions in the hypothalamus, a vital brain center. But these studies represent extreme circumstances—the lesions didn't appear when MSG was added in normal amounts to the animals' diets—so they don't really provide any information about human consumption of MSG.

In 1995, a panel of experts convened by the Food and Drug Administration concluded that MSG doesn't cause any long-term medical problems. It did confirm that some people have strong short-term reactions within a half hour of eating three grams or more in a meal—about six times the amount you're likely to get in a single serving. The experts also found that people with severe asthma may suffer bronchospasms six to twelve hours after ingesting MSG, and that some individuals may react strongly even to very small amounts.

I have seen enough cases to convince me that MSG sensitivity is real. And when I go to Chinese restaurants (or others that might use MSG), I always ask to have the food prepared without it. Check the labels of the processed foods you eat for MSG; the manufacturer is required to list it on the label. Free glutamate is also present in various flavorings: hydrolyzed vegetable protein, calcium caseinate, sodium caseinate, soy sauce, and autolyzed yeast. Check the label for these as well. I don't know of any antidote to MSG, but one study has suggested that people who react to it are deficient in vitamin B-6; when they were given extra B-6 as a regular part of the diet, their symptoms didn't recur.

Healing with Magnets?

Q:
A member of my family consulted a healer regarding her general health, and was given magnets in order to correct her magnetic field. She is to place the left foot on one magnet and the right foot on a different magnet every day. The healer told her that this will correct imbalances caused by strong electromagnetic fields such as the ones in New York's subway system. Is this use of magnets safe, and can it be beneficial?

A:
Magnet therapy is growing in popularity after a long history rooted in the ancient cultures of China, India, and Egypt. There are various theories on the effects of magnets on the body and all sorts of claims as to their power. Roger Coghill, a British scientist, theorizes that magnets affect the iron in red blood cells, improving the blood's oxygen-carrying ability. Others say magnets stimulate nerve endings and modify electrical processes in the body. They suggest that magnets can help counteract electromagnetic pollution from devices like microwave ovens and television sets (and the New York subway system, I suppose). Frankly, we don't know a lot about the positive or negative medical effects of magnets and magnetic fields. Researchers are just beginning to explore this area.

People use magnets to relieve pain, accelerate healing, and boost mental and physical energy. For example, to relieve a toothache, magnet devotees will place the north magnetic pole of a magnet against the cheek for fifteen to twenty minutes. Putting the north pole on the forehead between your eyebrows for ten minutes at bedtime is supposed to lead to better sleep after a few days.

A number of Japanese magnetic devices are available for relief of pain, such as the pain of arthritis. You can buy magnet insoles, magnet mattress pads, magnet car-seat covers, and small magnets to place on various parts of your body. I've met patients who swear by them, but I don't think we can assume that wearing magnets is necessarily healthful—or helpful. Also, these devices are quite expensive.

Some people say that while contact with a south magnetic pole is relaxing, contact with a north magnetic pole can be stimulating and might activate latent tumors or other disease processes. Until the new field of energy medicine really gets going, I think we'll have to experiment on our own and watch for results of studies as they appear. For an overview of the subject written by an enthusiast, look up *Discovery of Magnetic Health: A Health Care Alternative* by George J. Washnis and Richard Z. Hricak.

When to Get a Mammogram?

Q:
I'm totally confused by recent medical reports providing conflicting information about when women should go for mammograms. In your opinion, at what age should women start getting them on a regular basis?

A:
I'm not surprised by your confusion. Public health authorities are at odds over this question, and the debate isn't over yet. Meanwhile, women are left in the dark on how best to take care of themselves.

The issue in question is whether women in their forties should get routine mammograms to screen for breast cancer in its earliest stages. Very recently, the American Cancer Society issued new guidelines for mammograms, recommending that women in their forties have the cancer screening performed annually. Previous guidelines recommended mammograms every one to two years starting at age forty, and every year beginning at age fifty. The panel said that annual mammograms for women in their forties could save as many as 10,000 lives in the next five years.

According to Dr. Marilyn Leitch, an oncologist at the University of Texas Southwestern Medical Center, "The current average two-year interval between mammograms may be too long in this age group and their faster-growing cancers."

Just when a woman should begin mammography screening has been hotly debated since 1993, when the National Cancer Institute (of the National Institutes of Health) backed off its guideline that women should start the screenings at age forty. In 1996 the issue took on new significance with the appearance of mixed data about the benefits of screening women in their forties.

In my opinion, one of the most important things to keep in mind is that the effectiveness of a mammogram as a diagnostic technique depends entirely on the experience and skill of the person who reads it. Be sure to go to an expert. If you don't know whom to call, contact the American Cancer Society at 800 ACS-2345 (227-2345). It's also my experience that mammograms do pick up tiny cancers that if left until palpable would be much more serious and life-threatening. I know several women whose lives were saved by early detection of breast cancer after a mammogram.

The downside, of course, is the amount of radiation involved. As readers know, I am opposed to needless exposure to X-ray radiation. The ultimate conclusion of the NIH panel is that every woman needs to decide for herself whether to get a mammogram and at what age; this decision should be based on her family history and risk profile.

Do Marijuana Users Need Additional Vitamins?

Q:
What vitamins would you recommend to keep an otherwise healthy marijuana smoker in the best shape? I've heard that marijuana depletes certain vitamins in the body.

A:
If you use any drug (alcohol, amphetamines, barbiturates, cocaine, narcotics, or marijuana), I would recommend taking a B-complex supplement every day in addition to a basic antioxidant formula (see page 10).

This cocktail helps protect your immune and healing systems, giving your body an edge against all kinds of irritation, including that produced by smoking anything—marijuana or tobacco. Medical evidence for the beneficial effects of antioxidant vitamins and minerals keeps accumulating. In addition, drink plenty of water (everyone should drink six to eight glasses a day) and try to breathe fresh air as often as possible.

Latest on Melatonin?

Q:

What do you think of melatonin? Is 3 milligrams a normal dose?

A:

Melatonin is the first and only effective remedy for jet lag, and I recommend it for that purpose (it's even effective for west-to-east travel, which many people find harder). It's also useful as an occasional remedy for insomnia—especially for people working shifts—or for disturbed sleep cycles. If you go through periods where you're dead tired at 7 P.M. and then find yourself wide awake at, say, 11 P.M., melatonin might change your cycle, allowing you to go to sleep at a better time and sleep for the whole night. For these uses, taking melatonin for only one or two nights might be sufficient.

But evidence for melatonin's effects as an immune-booster and a chemical fountain of youth is lacking—popular books and articles notwithstanding. Because it is a brain hormone, secreted by the pineal gland, with very general effects on the body, I'm wary about recommending it for use on a regular basis over long periods of time.

You should also know that the quality of melatonin products on the market is uneven, and many dosage forms are too high. A 1-milligram tablet taken sublingually (under the tongue) is probably more than enough for any use. The best book on the topic is *Melatonin,* by Russel J. Reiter, Ph.D., and Jo Robinson.

Help for Migraines?

Q:
What is the best natural cure for migraine headaches?

A:
Migraines are very unpleasant, often putting people out of action for days at a time as well as frustrating doctors, who frequently find that their arsenal of medications doesn't do the job.

Allergy, hormonal fluctuations, stress, and heredity are all factors that trigger attacks. My recommendations include:

• Eliminate coffee and decaf (and other sources of caffeine). Once a patient is off caffeine, coffee can be used as a treatment. Drink one or two cups of strong coffee at the first sign of an attack, then go lie down in a dark room.
• Eliminate other dietary triggers like chocolate, red wine (sometimes white wine, too), strong-flavored cheeses, fermented foods (like soy sauce and miso), sardines, anchovies, and pickled herring.
• As a preventive, take feverfew herb (*Tanacetum parthenium*), a little plant related to the chrysanthemum. You can buy a plant at a local nursery—it's a common ornamental—and chew a few leaves a day (be warned: they don't taste great), or you can buy a standardized extract at any health food store. Read the label to make sure it has the nec-

essary active components, parthenolides, in it. One or two tablets or capsules a day will significantly reduce the frequency of migraines in many people. You can stay on feverfew indefinitely.

- Take a course of biofeedback training and learn how to raise the temperature of your hands. This will be a helpful tool to abort a headache at the start of an attack. To find a practitioner near you, look in the yellow pages or contact the Biofeedback Certification Institute of America.
- Use prescription medications sparingly. Try ergotamine to abort migraine attacks; it is a powerful constrictor of arteries that in order to work must be used at the first sign of an attack.
- Don't take Fiorinal on a regular basis. Many doctors prescribe it like candy to migraine sufferers without telling them that it contains an addictive downer (butalbital) and caffeine, as well as aspirin. Don't take prednisone or other steroids to prevent attacks; the potential dangers outweigh the benefits.

If you continue to have attacks, consider changing the way you think about your headaches. Migraine is like an electrical storm in the brain—violent and disruptive—but leading to a calm, clear state in the end. It's not so bad to have a headache once in a while; it actually can be a good excuse to drop routines, focus inwardly, and let stress dissipate. If you can come to accept the attacks in this way, they may occur less frequently.

Got (Way Too Much) Milk?

Q:
While growing up, I was told that milk was the essential drink for staying healthy. Today, the advertisements from milk producers boast of vitamins, minerals, and, of course, calcium, calcium, calcium. In nature, milk is given to infants as a special diet to help them grow quickly. But is it healthy for adults?

A:
Much of the information that you've received about milk as "the essential drink" does come from the dairy industry, which has a vested interest in seeing that as many people as possible become lifetime consumers of milk and milk products.

In nature, animals drink milk only in infancy. And in many parts of the world, people react with disgust to the idea of drinking milk as adults. Milk is indeed a source of protein and calcium that some people do well on. But many adults have problems with one or more of its components.

Except among people of northern European origin, 75 percent of adults can't digest lactose, the sugar in milk. As they grow out of childhood, they stop making the enzyme that breaks down lactose. When lactose-intolerant people drink milk, they experience immediate digestive upsets: gas, cramps, and diarrhea.

Butterfat, the fat in milk, is the most saturated fat in

the American diet. Cheese is often 70 percent—or more—fat by calories. Milk fat is a principal contributor to high cholesterol and atherosclerosis.

The protein in milk, casein, irritates the immune system in many people. This is the component of milk that stimulates mucus production as well. Casein is responsible for milk's association with conditions like recurrent ear infections in early life, eczema, chronic bronchitis, asthma, and sinusitis.

Most commercial milk also contains residues from drugs, hormones, and chemicals used to keep modern dairy cows producing abundantly.

I think most people should limit their intake of whole milk and the products made from it. Lactose-intolerant adults can eat cultured milk products (such as yogurt) now and then. To enjoy milk products occasionally without exposing yourself to so much fat, you can eat nonfat yogurt and mozzarella or other lowfat cheeses.

The dairy industry has done a great job convincing us that children are deprived without milk. I've kept my own five-year-old daughter off milk until recently. She has been remarkably healthy and has never had an ear infection.

I give her goat's milk, Rice Dream (which comes in different flavors), or a new product called DariFree. It's made from potatoes, and I think it's the best-tasting of the milk substitutes. The company has a toll-free information number: 800 275-1437. You should be aware that rice and potato drinks aren't protein-based. If you give any of these milk substitutes to your children, you'll also have to provide them with a different source of protein. (Soy milk does contain protein and is a good substitute for many people, but children are sometimes allergic to it.)

As for calcium, which helps regulate the nerves and muscles and is necessary for building strong bones, there are other ways to get it. Cooked greens (especially collards), molasses, sesame seeds, broccoli, and tofu are good sources.

Do Mosquitoes Love You?

Q:

Are there any natural ways to prevent getting mosquito bites? Once you've been unlucky enough to get bitten, are there any ways to stop the itch and swelling?

A:

Mosquitoes are definitely attracted to some people more than others. And some people react more strongly to mosquito bites than others. I'm no fan of chemical sprays like Off! and Cutter, because the active ingredient—Deet—feels nasty and is toxic.

You can try using one of the natural bug repellents that you'll find in health food stores. Frankly, though, I think these work only if the mosquitoes are not too populous, and if you apply the stuff very frequently.

Some friends swear by Skin-So-Soft, a bath oil made by Avon, which seems to offer some protection. Other ways to escape include going indoors at mosquito feeding time—usually at dusk—or wearing long-sleeve, loose-fitting clothing and tucking your pants into your socks. Black and white fabrics seem to attract the bugs. So all you downtown types might go for earth tones when in the country.

Once you're bitten, you can try a couple of things. I use a bit of red Tiger Balm dabbed on the bite to distract myself from the itching. Some people use aloe vera.

If you can reduce your allergic responsiveness through changes in your diet or mental attitude, mosquito bites may not bother you so much. Try eating garlic or reducing the protein in your diet. (High levels of protein can irritate the immune system, aggravating your reactivity.)

You may also want to try taking B-complex vitamins regularly during the summer months. Mosquitoes seem to find some people's blood a little less palatable after a few weeks of the supplements.

How Good Are Multivitamins?

Q:

I'd like your opinion on multivitamins. I'm in good health but often can't eat right. Is a good multi advisable? And if so, what should I look for? Is there any difference between different brands of the exact same vitamins? What's the best way to compare them?

A:

If you're not eating regularly, if your diet is not rich in fresh foods, and if you don't get plenty of fruits and vegetables, a multivitamin is an easy solution. It's better to take your vitamin cocktail in stages throughout the day, but I'm not opposed to taking your daily requirement all at once in one capsule, pill, or tablet after your biggest meal.

Some precautions: I would check the doses to make sure you're getting enough antioxidants. That would be 25,000 IU beta-carotene (preferably with other carotenes such as alpha-carotene, lutein, zeaxanthin, and lycopene), 400 IU of natural vitamin E (twice that much if you're over forty), and 2,000 milligrams of vitamin C, plus 200 micrograms of selenium a day. If not, take extra supplements to make up the difference.

It's also possible to get too much of some things in a multivitamin. You don't want more than 400 micrograms a day of folic acid, because then you risk masking a vitamin B-12 deficiency without added benefits from the folic acid. And make sure there's no iron in there if you're not a woman of menstruating age or a person with proven iron-deficiency anemia. Iron is an oxidizing agent that can promote cancer and heart disease, and the body has no way of eliminating excess amounts except through blood loss.

I don't think those vitamin packs are worth it. You can make up your own packs, if you want. Or if it's the convenience you're after, a multivitamin probably makes more sense.

In general, when shopping for the vitamins, there really aren't any buzzwords to look for. Just use the same common sense you might use when looking for a bottle of juice for lunch or the right flour for the bread you're baking. You want products free of dyes, preservatives, and nonessential additives. And you might as well check out the cheapest ones that are free of additives first.

Read the labels. See whether the vitamin is in the form you like—a big capsule, a soft gel capsule, or a tablet. Look at the dose, and make sure the cheapest isn't just a lower amount of the vitamin encased in the same number of tablets. And make sure you know the desired dose. For instance, you can buy a calcium supplement only to find out you need six tablets in order to get the dose you want. Once I got a B-50 B-complex home and then realized that it provided only 200 milligrams a day of folic acid—half the daily amount I recommend.

Generally, the difference between natural and synthetic vitamins is not important. An exception is vitamin E. Most of the vitamin E you see on store shelves is synthetic, noted as dl-alpha-tocopherol on the label.

Don't buy it. Instead, go for natural vitamin E, or d-alpha-tocopherol, combined with other tocopherols. Once you find a brand you like for a particular vitamin, stick with it.

You'll find there are enormous differences in pricing. I've gotten my best deals from Trader Joe's and some of the mail-order discount houses. It's worth doing some research to find reliable, low-priced sources. Two places to try are L&H Vitamins and The Vitamin Shoppe.

Knocked Out by Narcolepsy?

Q:

I was diagnosed with narcolepsy in 1989. However, the medication that I take—Dexedrine 5-milligram tablets two to four times a day—does not seem to be working as it once did. I take medication vacations on the weekends thinking that I will regain the same action that it once gave me. Are there any new meds on the market or alternative methods that you can suggest?

A:

Narcolepsy can be disabling. A neurological disorder, it makes people excessively sleepy at unpredictable times. People who have it may find it unbearably hard to stay awake during meetings or music recitals, while driving, during a conversation, whenever. Then, at night, it may be difficult to get restful sleep, in part because of vivid dreams.

You didn't mention the other condition that is linked with narcolepsy, called cataplexy, a sudden loss of voluntary muscle control without warning, usually triggered by strong emotion. People with cataplexy suddenly fall to the ground when anything makes them laugh or cry. Physical exercise, too, can cause the reaction, which usually lasts for just a few seconds.

About 1 in 2,000 people has narcolepsy. Lots of

times it's not diagnosed because people ignore their chronic sleepiness. There are also mild forms of cataplexy that cause people to drop objects or sit down suddenly.

The root cause of narcolepsy remains a mystery to neurologists. At Stanford University, researchers are studying a colony of Doberman pinschers, Labrador retrievers, and mixed breeds that have inherited the condition. They have linked the condition in dogs to a single gene that looks a lot like one of the human genes involved in managing the immune system. In humans, researchers found a gene called HLA-DR2 or HLA-DQwl in 98 percent of people with narcolepsy, but one-quarter of people without the condition also had HLA-DQwl, so there must be something else going on.

A neuroscientist at the University of California in Los Angeles has pinpointed a group of neurons that seem to fire at the wrong times, causing a mix-up of waking and sleeping states. People with narcolepsy can go on dreaming while they're awake, and when they're asleep, their brains may be operating as if they were awake. Some scientists think that cataplexy may happen when a person shifts into the paralysis of REM sleep during waking hours.

Doctors tend to prescribe tricyclic antidepressants like imipramine (Tofranil) or protriptyline (Vivactil) for cataplexy. They usually rely on stimulants to treat narcolepsy. But these can have significant side effects, such as anxiety, dependence, euphoria—and the one you describe, tolerance over time. Dexedrine is an old treatment and probably not the best choice anymore.

A company called Cephalon filed for regulatory

approval to sell one new drug, called modafinil (Provigil), in 1997. It's supposed to provide a substantial decrease in sleepiness with only minor side effects. Another possibility is yohimbine, from the bark of a West African tree, *Pausinystalia yohimbe*. In a small 1994 test, seven of eight men who took yohimbine were able to stay alert all day. One drawback is, again, the possibility of building tolerance. And some people have problems with stomach upset and flushing. But you might want to check with your doctor before taking either of these drugs.

As for nondrug treatments, it would be interesting to look at brain wave biofeedback. People can learn to condition fast-alert waves when they start to feel sleepy.

Some people also find several short catnaps (fifteen to twenty minutes) throughout the day to be a good coping strategy.

The National Sleep Foundation, at 202 785-2300, is collecting a database of people with narcolepsy, their family histories, and biological samples. They hope to connect patients with researchers for clinical studies. There is also a patient support group called the Narcolepsy Network.

How to Avoid the Nit Picking?

Q:

Any thoughts on treatment of head lice? We had a persistent case last year. Our pediatrician recommended Rid. I followed the directions to the letter, but the lice seem to be resistant. Only manual removal of lice and nits worked. If this happens again, do you know of an easier method?

A:

These tiny flat parasites are about the size of a sesame seed, and move from person to person by way of combs, hats, and personal contact. If you have kids in school, this might become a problem in your household. If you take a close look at the child's scalp with a magnifying glass, you can see little grayish-white eggs, or nits, attached to the hair shafts. You rarely see the adult lice.

Preparations like Rid and Kwell work to kill lice, but they are definitely toxic to people, too. The conventional treatment is 1 percent lindane (sold as Kwell) in a shampoo, cream, or lotion applied once a day for two days. Then you can comb the eggs out of the hair, row by row, using a fine-tooth comb. Lotions made with 0.5 percent malathion can also work. But both of these can be irritating and are flammable. Lindane is a cousin of DDT, and can harm the nervous system.

Organisms resistant to these treatments are increasing, and recurrence is common. It may be that you were seeing reinfection, or that enough of the eggs survived to make a comeback. Sometimes it's necessary to go back at the nits after they hatch (in about ten days). Also, you have to get rid of or properly clean all sources of the lice: combs, hats, clothing, rugs, even chair coverings (cleaning includes vacuuming, laundering, steam pressing, or dry cleaning).

For a safe treatment, I would consider Neem. Neem, derived from a tree in India, is sold in garden shops as a pesticide. You'll find it in stores that carry organic gardening supplies.

Another treatment people have found helpful is an herbal recipe consisting of 2 ounces of vegetable oil, 20 drops of tea tree oil, and 10 drops each of the following essential oils: rosemary, lavender, and lemon. Do a skin test on the inside of the elbow first, and wait several hours to make sure the strong oils don't irritate the skin. Leave the mixture on the infected head under a towel for an hour, then shampoo. You'll probably have to repeat this at least once to get rid of the next batch of hatched lice.

If you use any of these treatments, make sure your child's eyes are covered and that you apply the pesticide only to the head and neck.

Lice are awful for children because the itching is so severe. The easiest way to deal with the bugs is to avoid getting them, if at all possible (and sometimes that's difficult). Make sure your children don't share pillows, hats, combs, or hairbrushes with others. If there's an infestation at school, change the bedsheets often. Wash them in hot water and dry them in the dryer. Wash combs and brushes, and soak them in hot water for ten minutes. Check your children for head lice at least once a week, looking for nits behind the ears and above the neck.

Lice have made a major comeback in schools these days, so you have to stay on the lookout.

Just Say No to Laughing Gas?

Q:

Nitrous oxide—bad for the brain, or just clean fun?

A:

Nitrous oxide is also known as laughing gas. It got the name from traveling medicine shows and carnivals where the public would pay to inhale a minute's worth of the gas. People would laugh and act silly until the effect of the drug came to an abrupt end, when they would stand about in confusion. Yes, the good ol' days.

Nowadays, nitrous oxide is commonly used as a light general anesthetic for dental work and as a prelude to deeper anesthesia in surgery. It's also popular as a recreational drug to induce changes in consciousness or philosophical revelations, or just get hilariously intoxicated. The effects come on quickly and disappear just as fast.

Unfortunately, it isn't just clean fun. Nitrous oxide itself isn't bad for the brain, but unless you're careful in using it, you can deprive your brain of oxygen.

Some people breathe nitrous oxide straight out of tanks, a risky practice because you can asphyxiate yourself that way. Also, gas coming out of a pressurized tank is very cold and can cause frostbite of your nose, lips, or, most dangerously, larynx. Because of the anesthetic effects of the gas, you might not feel the damage until too late. The best way to avoid such dangers is to breathe nitrous oxide only from balloons— and only for a few minutes at a time.

Any way you breathe it, nitrous oxide can cause other serious injuries. People rapidly lose motor control under its influence and can fall over. So make sure you're sitting or lying down if you use it. It can also cause nausea and vomiting, particularly if you do it on a full stomach.

Regular use of nitrous oxide can impair fertility and interfere with the ability of the body to use vitamin B-12. A 1992 study published in the *New England Journal of Medicine* found that women exposed to high levels of nitrous oxide in their jobs (they were dental assistants) had a greater risk of infertility. Scientists speculate that the gas may interfere with the secretion of reproductive hormones. Interference with B-12 metabolism can result in damage to the bone marrow and nervous system. Loss of sensation in the feet and loss of balance may occur. I saw one patient, a man in his forties, who had developed severe pernicious anemia (vitamin B-12 deficiency) from breathing nitrous oxide on a regular basis and had those symptoms. It took a long time to clear up, even with regular vitamin B-12 shots.

Bothered by a Nosebleed?

Q:
Any cure for nosebleeding? What is the scientific name for it?

A:
Nosebleeds can look fairly dramatic because of all that bright red blood running down your face. But they're actually more of a bother than a medical problem— and definitely not life-threatening. Sometimes a nosebleed can be a symptom of something else, such as high blood pressure or a clotting disorder. But most often it's spontaneous and more likely to happen in winter than in any other season. When the lining of your nose dries out or there's a lot of sneezing or nose-blowing because you have allergies or a cold, the blood vessels close to the surface can rupture. This may happen when you're spending a lot of time in overheated rooms, or it may happen when someone punches you in the nose.

The first thing to do if you get a nosebleed is to blow your nose gently. Don't lean back. Instead, sit upright or lean your head slightly forward and pinch both nostrils. Hold them shut for five to ten minutes and breathe through your mouth. By plugging your nose, you stop the blood flow and allow the blood vessels to form a clot. If the bleeding hasn't stopped after ten minutes, spray some decongestant into your nose.

This shrinks the blood vessels and aids in repair. Then hold your nose again for ten minutes.

Another way to stop bleeding is to sniff a little bit of powdered yarrow. Yarrow, or *Achillea millefolium,* has a wonderful ability to stop bleeding.

If after twenty minutes you're still bleeding, it's best to go to a doctor to get the blood vessels sealed off with some silver nitrate solution. You'll also likely need professional help if you're taking blood thinners or large doses of aspirin.

Once you've stopped bleeding, don't blow your nose for a while or exert yourself—the bleeding could start up again.

If you live in a dry climate, one solution to regular nosebleeds is to use a humidifier in your home. Another option is to rub some liquid vitamin E in your nose. You can also try taking vitamin C as a supplement—at least 1,000 milligrams twice a day—since it decreases the fragility of small blood vessels. Another possibility is bilberry extract (from the European blueberry, *Vaccinium myrtillus*), which does the same thing.

By the way, the scientific name for nosebleed is "epistaxis."

What's Olestra All About?

Q:
I need info on olestra. What are the side effects? Does it take away nutrients from your system? I have heard that it flushes through the system and depletes vitamins. True?

A:
Olestra is a relatively new product that tastes and feels like fat but doesn't add fat or calories to the body because it's indigestible. The Center for Science in the Public Interest, a consumer group, asked the FDA to withdraw its approval of olestra because a study found that 20 percent of people who ate potato chips made with it had intestinal problems; for 3 percent of them, the problems were severe.

Olestra, manufactured by Procter & Gamble as Olean, is made with two natural products—sugar and vegetable oil. P & G replaces the glycerol in a normal fat with sucrose, then adds six, seven, or eight fatty acids instead of the three found in regular fat. What does this mean? Well, the resulting compound is too big to get into the bloodstream through the small intestine, so it really does flush through the system, as you say.

A 1-ounce serving of regular potato chips contains about 150 calories and 10 grams (90 calories) of fat.

Cooked in olestra, the same chips will contain about 70 calories and no fat.

The FDA approved olestra for use in potato chips, cheese puffs, crackers, and other salty snacks. P & G spent more than $200 million testing olestra to get it through regulatory scrutiny, but it is still under investigation for its long-term effects.

The studies found that olestra prevents absorption of vitamins A, D, E, and K, which hook onto the fat substitute and ride along as it passes through the intestine. The FDA required P & G to compensate by adding those vitamins to products containing olestra.

The fake fat also drags beta-carotene and other carotenoids along with it through the intestine and out of the body. Carotenoids may help prevent many kinds of cancer and other diseases, and some nutritionists have said they are concerned about the long-term impact of carotenoid loss due to olestra. Such questions are especially important since olestra could represent a significant change in the American diet, considering the quantities of fatty snacks people eat.

Other recorded side effects from olestra include bowel-function disruptions such as cramping, gas, diarrhea, and a problem euphemistically called "anal leakage."

The most pertinent question about olestra, though, is whether its benefits outweigh its potential hazards. Sugar substitutes haven't helped anyone lose weight. Whether fat substitutes will is not clear. I would say if you're going to consume olestra, do it moderately and cautiously until we have more information about it.

Abnormal Pap Smear?

Q:

Can an abnormal Pap smear be an indicator for any sexually transmitted diseases? And, related to that, why is it necessary to wait four months before going back to get another Pap smear?

A:

The aim of a Pap smear, named after Dr. George Papanicolaou, is to detect abnormal cells in the cervix, the doughnut-shaped entrance to the uterus. The idea is to identify cellular changes that can lead to cancer before they get out of control. The procedure is simple: a gynecologist uses a soft brush, called a cytobrush, to sample cells from just inside the cervical opening, and a small wooden or plastic spatula to gather cells from the outside. The cells are fixed on a slide and sent to a laboratory for analysis.

The Pap smear itself is not a diagnostic test for sexually transmitted diseases, but it can reveal conditions associated with them. In fact, most abnormal Pap slides result from infection with the human papillomavirus (HPV), not any malignancy. HPV is a very common sexually transmitted infection that causes venereal warts and is associated with cervical cancer. It's believed that you have to have HPV in order to develop cancer of the cervix. But HPV doesn't automatically lead to cancer—it just means you should be extra vigilant and get Pap smears yearly.

Most cervical cell changes discovered through a Pap smear return to normal on their own within a few months. That's why gynecologists will usually wait four months, then repeat the test. If the second test comes back clear, then it's best to repeat the smear a third time to make sure you get two negative tests in a row. False negatives occur often enough that I wouldn't be satisfied with just one negative result.

Cervical cancer is slow-growing, so a wait of four months shouldn't be a problem. If you want to be extra careful, or the second test comes back positive, you can have the abnormal tissue removed right away.

You should also know the risk factors for cervical cancer. These include infection with HPV, multiple childbirths, smoking, multiple sexual partners, first intercourse before age sixteen, and having a suppressed immune system. Whether or not any of these apply, however, I'd still recommend a Pap test once a year. The symptoms of cervical cancer include bleeding between periods or after intercourse, and abnormal vaginal discharge.

Women with cervical abnormalities tend to have weakened immune systems. They may suffer from low levels of vitamin A, B-complex vitamins—especially folic acid—and antioxidants. They may be experiencing extra stress. To help protect yourself against cellular changes in the cervix, the best thing to do is take good care of yourself and take my antioxidant cocktail (see page 10), plus a B-complex supplement that provides 400 micrograms of folic acid.

Poison on Your Peaches?

Q:
I eat lots of fruits and veggies, but I'm worried about pesticides and other contaminants. What do you think?

A:
You are right to be worried. Not so long ago, hundreds of people in eight states and Toronto got sick after eating berries (originally reported to be strawberries, but now known to have been raspberries) contaminated with *Cyclospora,* a parasite that causes diarrhea, vomiting, weight loss, fatigue, and muscle aches. Investigators have speculated that harvesting crews passed along the parasite because they had no toilet facilities in the field, nor any place to wash their hands.

As to pesticides, although organic produce is becoming much more widely available and cheaper to buy, it's still a hassle to get it in most parts of the country. So, if it's not organic, it's important to know what you're eating. Always peel and wash fruits and vegetables, even though you can't rely on these practices to remove all pesticides. First, you won't affect any "systemic chemicals" that are taken up in a plant's roots and spread through its tissues. Second, other chemicals adhere so tightly to the plant or penetrate so deeply that they can't be washed away. Canned or frozen foods aren't an alternative, because it's the same sprayed fruit that goes into the packaging.

So it's important for you to know which crops are likely to carry the heaviest pesticide residues. Fruits to watch out for include apples, peaches, Chilean grapes, Mexican cantaloupes, strawberries, apricots, and cherries. Vegetables, grains, and legumes that are commonly contaminated include spinach, cucumbers, bell peppers, peanuts, green beans, potatoes, and wheat. The wax on the outside of apples, cucumbers, and green peppers usually contains fungicides. You have to peel these foods to remove the toxins.

In general, beware of imported fruit, which usually isn't checked very well to see if growers have met U.S. pesticide standards, which are much stricter than those in many other countries.

Your best bets are not to eat these crops at all, to grow your own, or to eat organic. You can grow a surprising amount of food in a very small space, and enjoy the emotional and physical benefits of gardening besides. Also, watch for pesticide-free displays in your supermarket, and get to know the laws in your state that govern when produce can be labeled organic. You can join consumer action groups to demand safe foods and clear labeling. Finally, find out about subscription or community agriculture, in which groups of consumers contract with growers to provide regular deliveries of organically produced fruits and vegetables.

I encourage people to support the organic agriculture movement, which is finally gaining a lot of ground in this country.

Let's Get a Physical?

Q:

What would you recommend be included in an annual physical examination for a healthy forty-two-year-old? I've been trying to find information on this, but have been having trouble doing so.

A:

You don't say whether you're a man or a woman, so I'll answer for everyone. I'm not a believer in general physicals every year, but if you've never had a physical exam or haven't had one in a long while, get one. Even people in their twenties and thirties should get a complete check-up at some point as a baseline. General physicals become important as you enter your forties and fifties; then it makes sense to think about doing exams on a more regular basis.

The procedure should include a history—your description of your health history and any present problems—a physical examination by a doctor, and standard lab tests. It's important that you talk to your doctor about any concerns you have about your health. You might want to bring a list of questions. (In addition to physical symptoms, you should talk to your doctor about any emotional or psychological difficulties.) Remember, most doctors work under factory-like conditions these days, and you've got to make sure you get the attention you need. Be an assertive patient!

There are standard assessments that should be included in every physical exam and other tests that may be appropriate, depending on your medical history. Usually the doctor will start by recording your height, weight, pulse, and blood pressure, then check your heart, lungs, lymph nodes, and abdomen.

For anyone in his or her forties, the visit should include a rectal examination, plus a stool sample to test for blood. For women, the exam should include a breast and vaginal examination and a Pap smear (to check for cancer of the cervix). Women should have an annual breast exam, pelvic exam, and Pap smear.

There is also a standard battery of blood tests that should be done, including a complete blood count and an SMAC 20. I would also include a complete lipid panel to measure cholesterol and blood fats. Your urine should be sampled for testing, too.

Men over fifty should have a serum PSA (prostate specific antigen) test, which screens for prostate cancer, and an electrocardiogram (EKG). Women should have a mammogram at age forty.

Pained by Plantar Warts?

Q:
My nine-year-old daughter has a few hard, white spots on the soles of her feet. I thought they might be plantar warts, as she goes barefoot in her weekly karate classes, but I'm not sure. How can I tell? Is there anything else that could be causing these white spots? There are three small spots, on one foot only.

A:
Plantar warts are just warts on the bottom of the foot, which is called the plantar surface. Ta-da: plantar warts! And because you put the whole weight of your body on your feet every day, they often get inflamed and painful. Warts are caused by the human papillomavirus (HPV).

I'd guess your diagnosis is correct, but you can be sure by taking a closer look. Get a magnifying glass and see if these dots show the characteristic appearance of a wart, that is, not smooth and hard, but with a rough, corrugated surface. Usually there will be a soft center, with rough rings around it. You may also see little black dots in the warts, which are bits of coagulated blood. If the spots don't look like this, or grow progressively larger and more tender, your daughter could have foreign bodies, like splinters, lodged under her skin. Doctors put acid on warts, freeze them off, or use an electric spark to burn them. Earl Mindell, in his

Vitamin Bible, suggests applying 28,000 IU of vitamin E (from oil-base capsules) externally, one to two times a day, plus 400 IU (dry form) taken internally three times a day. But the best approach, especially in young people, is healing by suggestion. That would be my treatment of choice.

Children are especially good at visualizing warts away. You can go to a hypnotherapist or guided imagery therapist for help, but I'd give it a try on my own first. Work with your daughter to come up with an image that has an emotional charge for her. And encourage her to use it at least twice a day, especially on going to bed and on waking. One man I know got rid of a troublesome wart by imagining a steam shovel scraping away at it morning and night. Maybe your daughter will want to imagine applying some of her martial arts techniques against the intruder. Working with mental imagery is a good way to mobilize your body's healing powers.

Eyeing Plastic Surgery?

Q:

I am thinking about having cosmetic surgery on my eyelids. I am only in my late twenties, but I have to do it because my eyelids really drag down. I don't know what I will look like afterward; all I can imagine is how horrific I am going to look with the stitches in. I have asked the plastic surgeon for some pictures, but he says he doesn't have any. What can I do about this anxiety, and the shock I will get when I see my eyes like that?

A:

First, please don't agree to have cosmetic surgery without really thinking it through carefully—not just about what it may look like along the way and afterward, but also about what you expect from it and why you want it. Be sure you really want this procedure. Ask your surgeon to explain in detail all the things that can go wrong. Find out what results the surgery can and can't give you. If your surgeon can't or won't tell you, look for a different one. I've written before about the importance of being an assertive patient; it is especially important when you are considering elective surgery. The cost for upper and lower lids can be as much as $7,000, and that won't be covered by your insurance provider.

As for your immediate concerns, you're right: you

have to be prepared for the week or two after surgery when you'll look worse than you did before it. It will take five to eight weeks until you're completely healed. A good resource for anyone considering plastic surgery is Diana Barry's *Nips & Tucks: Everything You Must Know Before Having Cosmetic Surgery*. Barry covers everything from eyelid surgery to collagen injections and postmastectomy breast reconstruction.

Other, more invasive procedures—like face-lifts—can take even more time to heal fully (and can leave you with permanent side effects). I've seen some very good results from cosmetic surgery. But I've also seen a number of cases where faces ended up looking very unnatural, with the skin appearing stretched, for example.

I don't know if you smoke. People who smoke tobacco are at higher risk for complications from cosmetic surgery, because they have decreased blood circulation in the skin. If you can't quit altogether, your surgeon will suggest stopping ten days before surgery, and for a week post-op. That's the minimum.

I also have to say that all this sounds premature. You said you're in your twenties, which is very young to be considering cosmetic surgery. Ask yourself a few basic questions before you do anything else. Why aren't you happy with yourself as you are? Is your unhappiness with your eyelids reflective of a larger dissatisfaction with yourself? Does your decision to change your eyelids rest on what other people have been telling you about your appearance? Maybe there are ways other than surgery for you to become happier. How about talking over the possibilities with a counselor before going further?

How to Soothe the Poison Ivy Itch?

Q:
What is the best way to cure or alleviate the itchiness of poison ivy or poison oak?

A:
About half the population is susceptible to poison ivy, poison oak, and poison sumac, all members of the genus *Rhus*. The itching, blistering reaction you get from these plants is caused by a T-cell response to urushiol, the allergenic component of the oil the plants produce. If you think you're one of the lucky ones who happen to be immune, beware: allergy to these plants can come and go quite suddenly.

The reaction usually occurs thirty-six to forty-eight hours after contact and lasts for about two weeks. You won't spread the rash by scratching the blisters, but it can spread internally around the body and surface in unexpected places.

Of course, the best defense against this family of plants is to learn how to recognize its members and avoid them. They can grow as shrubs or vines, and can be spotted by their characteristic clusters of three leaflets. The leaves can be shiny green, red-green, or red, depending on the season. If you do touch one of the plants, wash the oil off with soap and water within twenty to thirty minutes of contact. After that, the oil soaks into the skin. Watch and wash your pets, too.

One common way to get the rash is to touch a dog that has rubbed against a plant and picked up oil on its coat.

Tecnu sells a very effective over-the-counter product that will remove the oils of poison oak, ivy, or sumac from the skin up to twenty-four hours after contact. The company also makes a protective lotion that you can put on your skin before you go out in the woods. These are the best preventive products I've found.

The absolute best treatment I know for poison ivy is to get in the shower and run hot water—as hot as you can stand—over the affected area for five to ten minutes. This seems counterintuitive, because it will increase the itching. But after a few minutes, the nervous circuits seem to get overloaded and the itching stops for a long time. If you conscientiously repeat the hot water treatment whenever the itching returns, the whole reaction completes its cycle rapidly and your skin will return to normal.

While hot water works better than anything, you also can use calamine lotion as a topical treatment if you wish. I strongly recommend against taking oral prednisone or other steroids unless there are very severe symptoms, such as fever or difficulty in urinating. Don't use topical steroids, either. Steroids are toxic drugs that should be saved for serious conditions, not minor ones, since they suppress the immune system.

SOS for PMS?

Q:
I am a victim of premenstrual syndrome (PMS). It has gotten progressively worse in the past year, I'd say. My moods are so extreme, it is difficult for me to be around other humans. I go from being filled with rage and hostility to feeling anxious and scared for no reason, to sobbing uncontrollably at the drop of a hat. I recently went on the Pill, which has made my cycle more predictable, but I'm still an emotional basket case. My boyfriend is ready to kill me. Please help.

A:
Many male doctors consider PMS an imaginary condition, and some feminists believe it's a construct of the male establishment. Nevertheless, many women suffer severe physical discomfort, plus the mood swings you mention, just before the onset of menstruation. Common symptoms include depression, tension, anger, difficulty concentrating, lethargy, changes in appetite, and a feeling of being overwhelmed. These can be accompanied by breast tenderness, headache, fluid retention, and joint or muscle pain. PMS's effects may begin around the time of ovulation, then diminish during menstruation or just after.

It is possible to ease the severity of PMS or even eliminate it entirely. First, I'd suggest removing all caffeine—including chocolate—from your life. Many women crave chocolate just before menstruation and say it acts as an antidepressant. But it can be addictive and can have a powerful effect on moods, energy cycles, and sleep patterns. Caffeine adds to nervous tension and increases your heart rate. (So beware of using caffeine or chocolate as a spiritual or emotional salve.) Also avoid all polyunsaturated vegetable oils, which can promote inflammation.

Next, you should exercise regularly. I would suggest thirty minutes of some sustained aerobic activity five days a week. Besides giving a sense of strength and well-being, and increasing the flow of oxygen to all organs, exercise helps to regulate your hormone levels.

Third, take a supplement of evening primrose oil or black currant oil, two capsules two or three times a day. Both supplements supply an unusual fatty acid called gamma linolenic acid (GLA), an effective anti-inflammatory agent. (GLA also promotes healthy skin, hair, and nails.) Try this for at least two months and continue if you feel better. I also would take supplements of calcium and magnesium, preferably 1,200 to 1,500 milligrams of calcium citrate at bedtime, and half that amount of magnesium. These may ease menstrual cramps.

You might experiment with several herbs that have a good track record with PMS. The first is dong quai, a Chinese remedy made from the root of *Angelica sinensis*, in the carrot family. It acts as a general tonic for the female reproductive system in much the same way that ginseng works for men. You can try two capsules twice a day for several months to see how it affects you. Another possibility is vitex, or chaste tree (*Vitex agnus-castus*), in the same dosage. It helps regulate the female reproductive cycle. Try these one at a time to assess their benefit.

As a general tonic for your mind, body, and moods, experiment with deep breathing and other relaxation techniques. It may also be helpful to analyze which symptoms you are feeling and when. Try listing the symptoms that bother you most, then recording when you experience them during the month. This can help you be aware of what to expect each month, and also clarify which symptoms are actually tied to your menstrual cycle and which might have another cause.

Radiation Dangers from Household Appliances?

Q:

I see a lot of news about radiation emitted by every-thing from cellular phones to radios to electric blan-kets. What are your opinions regarding the risks from these devices?

A:

Much has been written about the dangers of electric clock radios, electric blankets, heating pads, and hair dryers. All of these appliances generate electromag-netic fields that can disrupt delicate body control systems, possibly increasing the risk of cancer and weakening immunity. I wouldn't keep an electric clock radio near my head, and I wouldn't use any of these appliances on a regular basis. The best source of information about household radiation is *Cross Currents* by Robert O. Becker, M.D.

As for cellular phones, most of the scientists and all the manufacturers say there's nothing of concern here, despite the media furor. I have seen ads for shields that you can slip over the phone to block any radia-tion. If you're worried, do that.

Microwave ovens are generally safe; they rarely leak radiation, unless damaged. But they can alter the chemistry of protein foods cooked in them for long periods of time as well as drive foreign molecules into food wrapped in plastic wrap or cooked in plastic containers.

(Some cooking tips: Use microwaves for defrosting and quick heating, rather than long cooking of main dishes. Always use glass or ceramic containers to cook in. Never use plastic wrap during cooking.)

Everyone I've spoken to says that the new generation of computer monitors presents little risk or hazard. Most of the radiation comes out of the back—a fact you should be aware of. I used to use a computer monitor shield, but with a more recent model I don't. Because radiation falls off exponentially with distance, it never hurts to put a little more distance between you and the source.

Is Radon
Really Dangerous?

Q:

*How dangerous is radon? We have lived for over fif-
teen years in a house that has from 17 to 28 picocuries
per liter of radon in the basement, where our family
room, computer room, and playroom are located. My
husband doesn't want to spend the money to get rid of
the radon.*

A:

Radon is a natural radioactive element produced by
the decay of radium in the Earth's crust. It's an odor-
less, colorless gas that seeps out of the earth, more
commonly in some places on the planet than others. It
sometimes enters the basements of houses through
cracks and pipes and becomes trapped there, concentrated in the air we breathe.

Radon is strongly carcinogenic, and is believed to
be the second leading cause of lung cancer—after
cigarette smoking. It may account for as many as
30,000 deaths a year in the United States. Radon is
dangerous, but I don't think anyone can say exactly
how dangerous. You can have the air in your house
tested for radon, but if there's a high level, it's not
clear what you should do.

Check with your regional office of the Environmental Protection Agency. Those folks can tell you how
serious your problem may be and which ventilation

systems work best. You also can get information on test kits and ways to reduce gas levels through the National Safety Council's National Radon Hotline at 800 767-7236.

You can install an exhaust system, which may remove the radon from the air coming into the basement. You can also cover and seal drains, pipes, and cracks in the foundation, where the radon could be leaking in. If the level stays at 4 picocuries per liter (pCi/L) or higher and you are concerned, you may want to move to another house. Obviously, that's easier said than done.

The bottom line: Radon is dangerous, and if there's a significant level of it in your house, I think you and your husband should spend the money to do something about it.

Red Wine for a Healthy Heart?

Q:

What are the pros and cons of drinking red wine?

A:

The wine industry has benefited tremendously from reports that moderate drinking of red wine can lower the risk of coronary heart disease. After *60 Minutes* reported on the "French Paradox" in 1991, sales of cabernet and merlot soared.

The French Paradox was first discovered when epidemiologists tried to explain the lower-than-expected death rates from heart disease in France in spite of a high-fat, high-cholesterol diet. Various studies followed that showed an association between drinking red wine and a heart attack risk that was 25 to 40 percent lower. *60 Minutes* followed up with a report from the Copenhagen City Heart Study of 13,000 people over ten years: the researchers had concluded that teetotalers had twice as much risk of dying from heart disease as people who drank wine every day.

The exact mechanism isn't known, but the most popular explanation credits the red pigments in grape skins. These pigments belong to a family of compounds called proanthocyanidins, which are powerful antioxidants that may protect arteries from circulating cholesterol. If this is the primary action, you could get the same benefits from drinking red grape juice or

eating enough red and purple fruit. In fact, more recent research makes red grape juice look even more
protective than red wine.

The tannins in red wine as well as the alcohol can
keep platelets in the blood from clumping together
and triggering a heart attack. Plus, studies have found
that any alcohol can raise levels of HDL—the good
form of cholesterol that prevents arterial damage.

But let's not forget that alcohol is toxic to the liver
and nervous system. The French have a higher risk of
liver disease. Most wines also contain a variety of additives, such as sulfites, which may be unhealthy. If
you're going to be a regular wine drinker, I'd recommend moderation. I'd also look for organic products.
Both domestic and imported organic wines of good
quality are becoming more available.

I don't drink red wine because it gives me a stuffy
nose and a morning-after sour stomach—probably
reactions to additives or constituents other than alcohol. Red wine is a common allergen that can trigger migraine headaches as well as nasal and gastric
disturbances.

Find the Right Shrink?

Q:

The psychiatrist I was seeing retired after just three visits, and I began to see another doctor a month ago. My question now is, is it better to see a psychiatrist or a psychoanalyst? One of my main problems is dependency. I can't seem to make decisions without the approval or support of someone. I was told that besides giving you Xanax for anxiety, a psychiatrist tends to listen more and let you figure out your own problems, and an analyst becomes more involved in discussion with the patient. Which is better for me?

A:

The bottom line for mental-health care is really a matter of what you can afford, how much time you want to devote to the problem, and, most important, the chemistry between you and the counselor you choose.

Managed care has changed the way mental-health services are provided. Because of time constraints and limits on the number of visits allowed, more mental-health providers now lean toward drug therapy instead of problem-solving sessions. Most health plans cover only a few visits a year, and will pay no more than $50,000 in mental-health care over a lifetime. On first glance that may seem like a lot, but the dollar amount also encompasses hospitalization for serious mental illnesses, which is expensive.

Psychiatrists are M.D.s, and they can prescribe medication. Their medical training has concentrated on the treatment and prevention of mental, emotional, and behavioral disorders. Psychoanalysts are a special subclass of psychiatrists with additional training who subscribe to Sigmund Freud's theories and try to help you become aware of unconscious drives that affect behavior. Generally, the psychoanalyst sits out of sight while the patient reclines on a couch, recounting dreams, describing childhood incidents, and free-associating. Many try to inject themselves as little as possible into the unfolding of the patient's unconscious. Psychoanalysis is very time- and cost-intensive, and is sharply declining in popularity.

Psychologists and licensed clinical social workers engage in interactive counseling, helping the patient unravel the interaction between buried drives, past history, and physical and social environment; often, they turn to dreams and childhood memories as tools. More and more, the lines are becoming blurred between the different specialists. Managed care is encouraging streamlined approaches to all these interventions.

There are many subspecialties within each of the fields. Your best bet is to try out several people and see with whom you feel most comfortable. Ask them about the theories they use, the political ideologies they may apply, what they charge, what health plans they accept, and anything else that seems important to you. Ask what sessions with them will be like, and how long they think treatment may take.

It may be that you should be on medication, though I wouldn't want you to jump to that conclusion because you feel anxiety. There are other effective methods to relieve anxious feelings, and only someone who sees you in person and talks with you at length can help you decide what's best. Even then, it may require some experimentation.

Xanax, or alprazolam, is an addictive drug that can interfere with mental function, so you may want to consider alternative treatments before you start taking it. A natural remedy for anxiety is tincture of passionflower (*Passiflora incarnata*), which is mildly relaxing. The dose is one dropperful in a little water up to four times a day, as needed. Tincture of valerian (*Valeriana officianalis*) is more powerful—use 10 to 15 drops in water up to four times a day as needed. I also recommend trying my relaxing breathing exercise (see page 233).

Is Rolfing Better than Massage?

Q:
I'd like to know your opinions on Rolfing and if you think it is a more beneficial form of massage than others. Thanks.

A:
Rolfing is not simply massage. It's a form of body work intended to restructure the connective tissue, or fascia. Basic Rolfing consists of ten intensive sessions in which the practitioner applies firm—even painful—pressure with the fingers and elbows to specific parts of the body. For people who are open to Rolfing, it can be a great way to get more in touch with your body and change long-standing problems of bad posture and chronic pain (like back pain). Rolfing can also release repressed emotions as well as diminish habitual muscle tension. If you want to make some kind of change in your life and work on your body, you might consider Rolfing. For a referral in your area, contact the Rolf Institute (see Other Resources, page 294).

What's Up with RU-486 (the Abortion Pill)?

Q:
Was RU-486 approved, and where is it available?

A:
RU-486, the French abortion pill, is still making its way through an obstacle course into the U.S. drug system—although it's now close to approval. The Food and Drug Administration recently said it would allow sale of the drug, pending more information on how RU-486 will be labeled and manufactured. There will be certain rules to ensure its safety. For example, doctors who prescribe it must meet certain requirements, and women who take it must live within an hour of emergency treatment in case something goes wrong.

I'm happy to see this drug finally become available as an option for women who want abortions. Known chemically as mifepristone, it's vastly superior to the methods available now. Still, RU-486 should not be taken lightly. It requires three steps. First, the woman takes 600 milligrams of RU-486 to end the pregnancy. It's 95.5 percent effective when used within the first seven weeks. Then she must take another drug to induce contractions in the uterus to expel the fetus. Finally, she must go back in for an exam to make sure the pregnancy has been aborted.

Using this drug is much less traumatic than under-going surgery. The side effects are similar to those of a spontaneous miscarriage: bleeding, cramps, nausea, and fatigue. Serious complications are rare. In clinical trials in the United States, 4 out of 2,100 women needed a blood transfusion because of uncontrolled bleeding.

Women began using RU-486 in France in 1988. Protests by antiabortion groups were so venomous, however, that manufacturer Roussel-Uclaf suspended distribution. Almost immediately, the French Minister of Health stepped forward and ordered the company to sell the drug in the interest of public health. I've heard that about 200,000 women have used the drug in Europe—it's approved in France, the United Kingdom, and Sweden. In the United States, the Bush administration was not so open-minded. It banned the import of RU-486. Clinton lifted the prohibition in 1993, and Roussel-Uclaf gave the rights for the drug to a nonprofit research institution in New York, the Population Council, which began clinical trials here to test safety and effectiveness.

An FDA advisory committee recommended approval for RU-486 in July 1996; then the FDA announced in September 1996 that it was ready to approve the drug, which will probably be renamed in the United States.

The clinical trials have been completed, but there appear to be several outstanding issues to be resolved before RU-486 is available in the United States. Meanwhile, you can keep up with RU-486's progress by checking with the National Abortion and Repro-ductive Rights Action League and the Planned Parent-hood Federation (800 230-PLAN).

Sauna Making
You Sweat?

Q:
*I've heard totally varied opinions on the benefits/
hazards of saunas and steam baths. What's your
opinion?*

A:
To me, the benefits far outweigh the hazards. If you're
in reasonable health, the benefits of a sauna or steam
bath are great. If you have high blood pressure or
heart disease, saunas may be good for you, but you'll
want to be cautious; check with your physician first,
and go slow. And with either of these conditions, it's
not a good idea to jump right into cold water afterward, as Finns do.

When you take a sauna, the heat pumps up blood
circulation near the skin and stimulates sweating. The
Finns say a proper sauna elicits about a quart of sweat
per hour. I generally encourage sweating, because it
helps the body rid itself of unwanted materials. In me-
dieval times, healers relied on sweat baths to cure illnesses, and priests used them to chase away evil
spirits.

American physicians usually warn pregnant women
not to take steam baths or saunas. A study published
in 1992 in the *Journal of the American Medical Association* found some association between neural tube
defects and heat exposure from saunas, hot tubs,

and fever during the first three months of pregnancy. (Neural tube defects include anencephaly and spina bifida, both disastrous fetal abnormalities.) The biggest problem was posed by hot tubs, which pregnant women should definitely approach with caution.

Interestingly, though, in Finland it's not uncommon for doctors to give the OK on saunas from conception all the way up to the day of delivery—and there, neural tube defects are very low. In fact, in Finland saunas were once a traditional place for childbirth. It's worth noting that Finnish women tend to stay in the sauna for six to twelve minutes, and they shorten that time during pregnancy. Also, even though they feel very hot, saunas raise the body's core temperature insignificantly compared to hot tubs.

Finnish saunas are different from most U.S. versions—unless these are run by Scandinavians. In Finland, saunas are usually heated by a wood stove. First there's a dry phase that can get hotter than 200° F. Then the participants splash water on the stove and spend some time in the steam. Many U.S. saunas employ an electric stove, which you can't put water on. So you're just exposed to dry heat, which I, for one, find irritating to my respiratory passages. Some saunas in health clubs are set to a lukewarm temperature. Turn up the heat.

Even if you're in a very hot steam bath or sauna, it's mostly the temperature of the surface of your body that goes up. As it does so, blood vessels dilate, and circulation increases in the skin. As resistance to blood flow through your veins and capillaries drops, your blood pressure goes down. Then your heartbeat increases to keep blood pressure normal.

Finns always follow a sauna with a plunge into cold water. This is incredibly refreshing and enjoyable. Then you relax.

The main risk of a sauna is staying in too long and fainting from overheating. People who are most susceptible are those with heart disease and those who have been using drugs or alcohol. It isn't a good idea to combine alcohol and other drugs with saunas or hot tubs. Also, be sure you drink plenty of water, to replace the water you're losing. Children should not use saunas or hot tubs without supervision.

By the way, the correct pronunciation is *sow-na,* not *saw-na.*

Seeking News on Selenium?

Q:
I've been reading a lot about selenium in the newspaper these days. Can it really prevent cancer?

A:
The recent study about selenium that came out of the University of Arizona caused quite a stir. For a long time, people have believed that selenium protects against cancer, heart ailments, and other diseases. But studies on the subject were in disagreement. So the Arizona Cancer Center at the University of Arizona in Tucson, where I teach, planned a randomized trial to study the ability of selenium supplements to protect against two skin cancers: basal cell carcinoma and squamous cell carcinoma. Dr. Larry Clark and a team of researchers recruited 1,312 patients from the eastern coastal plain of the United States, where selenium levels in the soil and crops are low, and skin cancer rates are high. All of the patients had a history of the disease. Half of the group received sugar pills every day for an average of 4.5 years, and the other half took 200 micrograms of selenium in supplement form each day.

Clark found that the selenium supplements didn't have any effect on skin cancers. But halfway through the study, the researchers decided to look at other types of cancers and cancer mortality in general. At the end of the study, they had some dramatic results. The people who had taken selenium had 63 percent fewer prostate cancers, 58 percent fewer colorectal cancers, and 46 percent fewer lung cancers than the rest of the group. Overall, there were 39 percent fewer new cancers among those taking selenium. And altogether, half as many died from their cancer. The selenium seemed to be so beneficial, the researchers stopped the blinded phase of the trial early.

There are several possible mechanisms for the protective effect of selenium. Selenium activates an enzyme in the body called gluthathione peroxidase that protects against the formation of free radicals—those loose molecular cannons that can damage DNA. In this situation, selenium may work interchangeably (and in synergy) with vitamin E. In test tube studies, selenium inhibited tumor growth and regulated the natural life span of cells, ensuring that they died when they were supposed to instead of turning "immortal" and hence malignant. Because of this particular action, the University of Arizona researchers say that selenium could be effective within a fairly short time frame.

There were some weaknesses in this study, among them the fact that few women were included. Because the results are not consistent with those of other studies (using lower doses), the researchers and other cancer specialists are calling for further randomized trials before any national recommendations are made about selenium supplementation.

I'm all for that. But in the meantime, I will continue to take my 200 micrograms of selenium a day—the same dose used in the study—and I suggest that you do, too. Excess selenium has been associated with toxicity, so don't go overboard. If you're not fond of popping pills, you can get 120 micrograms of selenium in just one Brazil nut. Buy the shelled kind—they're grown in a central region of Brazil where the soil is richest in the mineral. Other good sources are tuna fish, seafood, wheat germ, and bran.

A Proven Sex-Drive Enhancer?

Q:

Is there anything I can take to boost my sex drive? I'm female.

A:

Of course, people have been asking this question for centuries. Curiously enough, a proven sex-drive enhancer for women is the male hormone testosterone. Women produce their own testosterone, and reputable scientific studies show that tiny additional amounts can increase libido dramatically. One testosterone product, formulated for women in menopause, is called Estratest; it also contains estrogen. If you're interested in trying it, consult a gynecologist.

An herbal possibility for women is the Mexican plant damiana (*Turnera diffusa*), which has a reputation as a female aphrodisiac. Not that much is known about it, but you can find damiana preparations in health food stores. Again, follow dosage recommendations on the label. Whichever of these appeals to you, try it for a few months and see what it can do for you. If it works, great. If not, there's no point in continuing the treatment.

But before spending money on substances like these, you might want to consider other ways to boost sexual energy. Both physical and mental well-being are important to healthy sex. Think about the interplay of emotional charge, mental imagery, and body responses associated with sex. Hypnotherapy and guided imagery therapy can help you make the most of the mind-body connection in overcoming sexual problems. Many experts, myself included, say the greatest aphrodisiac is the human mind.

Cancer-Killing Sharks?

Q:

What do you know about cancer patients using shark cartilage? How does it work to help treat the cancer?

A:

Shark cartilage has become popular as an arthritis treatment and a therapy for cancer and AIDS. I haven't seen any good scientific evidence that it works, just anecdotal reports and suggestive laboratory studies. The theory is that shark cartilage contains substances that inhibit the proliferation of new blood vessels that tumors need in order to continue to grow. Mainstream scientists have isolated several compounds from shark tissue, notably squalamine, that do have this effect. But the shark antitumor substances they are investigating aren't found in the cartilage. Furthermore, even if there are beneficial substances in the cartilage, I'm not convinced the commercial capsules provide them in a form the body can absorb.

Most scientists object strongly to the intense promotion and commercialization of shark cartilage because there is so little evidence of its efficacy. Meanwhile, its popularity has helped decimate shark populations.

When considering alternative treatments for cancer, it's wise to seek good published data on outcomes from their use. If you can't find published data, ask to see statistical data from providers. Look particularly for any risk of toxicity or harm. And finally, ask to talk with patients who have undergone the alternative therapy. If you have cancer, it is important to work to improve overall health and resistance on all levels. A book on alternative cancer therapies I recommend to my cancer patients is *Choice in Healing,* by Michael Lerner.

Dangers of Silicone Implants?

Q:

I have never heard you speak on what women who have breast implants can do to help rid their bodies of the silicone gel. Many of us have developed multiple problems and are in a daily search for help. Any and all information would be greatly appreciated and shared with many.

A:

Women with side effects from breast implants often get hopeless prognoses from doctors, or else get treated as if their problems were imaginary. Medical literature does not support the existence of silicone disease, but it is obvious to me that women who have had silicone in their bodies may suffer from a variety of auto-immune reactions. The Food and Drug Administration put a halt to silicone implants in 1992 because of concerns about their safety.

I don't think it's a great idea to have silicone in the body, so if you've experienced any problems, I'd recommend having the breast implants removed. It's a tougher question if you're not having problems. If the implants are undamaged and intact, you're probably okay—and it may not be worth the trauma to have them removed. On the other hand, the implants can develop slow leaks, with complications showing up later. One sign of a problem is your breast becoming hard. An FDA panel estimated in 1992 that up to 6 percent of silicone implants rupture. If you're unsure—or just concerned—about the status of your implants, talk to your doctor; he or she can detect abnormalities by ultrasound mammography.

I don't know of any way to remove the silicone that may have leaked into your tissues. But I have seen great improvement in women who had the implants removed and then followed a program to improve their general health.

If you're experiencing problems, here are some steps you should take:

- Eat a low-protein diet, eliminate milk and milk products, and cut back on meat and other foods of animal origin.
- Avoid polyunsaturated oils.
- Eat fish and organically grown fruits, vegetables, and grains.
- Take antioxidant vitamins and minerals.
- Exercise regularly.
- Practice relaxation techniques and experiment with visualization, psychotherapy, and hypnotherapy.
- Consider traditional Chinese medical treatment or Ayurvedic medicine.
- Try ginger, which has an anti-inflammatory effect, as do feverfew and turmeric.

If you're experiencing autoimmune arthritis, I recommend one to two capsules of powdered, dried ginger twice a day, or one to two capsules of freeze-dried feverfew leaves twice a day. You can take turmeric in the form of curcumin (the active component, which happens to give turmeric its yellow pigment) in 400- to 600-milligram doses three times a day.

Could It Be Skin Cancer?

Q:
I've had a small, scab-like sore on my thigh for fifteen to twenty years. I suspect skin cancer. Is it really dangerous to ignore it? How fast does skin cancer grow, and how does it grow?

A:
Skin cancers are the most common form of cancer, and their incidence is climbing dramatically. The number of cases of melanoma—the deadliest form of skin cancer—alone grew by 21 percent in the past decade.

People are also getting better at spotting skin cancer, and that's very good news, because early treatment cures 95 percent of people with the disease. That's why it's important to pay attention to the kind of sore you've described.

Any sore that doesn't heal should be examined by a dermatologist. And even though you've had this one for such a long time, it's possible that it may have changed without your noticing. There's really no hard-and-fast rule for how quickly skin cancers grow. Some grow very slowly; others don't. In general, a sore that doesn't heal is a cause for concern. Only a medical professional can tell you what to do about it.

When checking yourself for signs of skin cancer, you should look for changes in freckles or moles and any new bumps or nodules. Are any moles larger than the diameter of a pencil eraser? Are they of mixed colors (especially including black)? Are their borders irregular? Do the areas around them look inflamed or pale? Are they getting bigger? Are they scaly, scabby, or do they fail to heal after a minor injury? If you answer yes to any of these questions, it doesn't necessarily mean the moles or other areas are cancerous, but it does mean they deserve examination.

The risk of melanoma is particularly high in people who have family histories of the disease, and in those who've experienced blistering sunburns before age twenty. Everyone should wear sunscreen every day (SPF-15, at least), cover up with long-sleeve, tight-weave clothing, and stay indoors or in the shade when the sun is highest in the sky and in the months around the summer solstice.

If you start taking these kinds of precautions now, you can dramatically reduce the chance of developing skin cancer later in life.

Commit to Quit Smoking?

Q:
I know I should quit. I just can't seem to. I desperately need help.

A:
Many smokers stare at themselves in the mirror, asking, "How do I quit?" It's hard. Tobacco, in the form of cigarettes, is the most addictive drug in the world— right up there with crack cocaine. There are two reasons for this: Nicotine is one of the strongest stimulants known, and smoking is one of the most efficient drug-delivery systems. Smoking actually puts drugs into the brain more directly than intravenous injection.

In the early part of this century, cigarette smoking was accepted, and was even considered healthy and glamorous. It was thought to promote mental acuity, efficiency, and relaxation. It is true that one of the "benefits" of smoking is a brief relief of internal tension; unfortunately, within twenty minutes the tension is back stronger than before, and the brain demands another fix.

Low-tar, low-nicotine cigarettes offer no great advantages. People tend to smoke more of them, or inhale more deeply to get the same amount of nicotine. Pipes and cigars, if the smoke is not inhaled, do not cause lung cancer and emphysema, but they do increase the risk of oral cancer (as do snuff and chewing tobacco).

I feel so strongly about the health risks of smoking that I will not accept patients who are users unless they are willing to try to quit. Many programs can help you: acupuncture, hypnotherapy, and support groups. There are also a slew of new devices on the market—nicotine patches and gum, for instance—that work for some. None of these methods works reliably for everyone. Most successful quitters do it on their own after one or more unsuccessful attempts. Going "cold turkey" also seems to work better than gradually cutting down.

Don't get discouraged. If you can't quit today, you may be able to tomorrow. Motivation is the key, and it can come only from you. Remember: You get credit for every attempt you make. In fact, the best predictor for success is making attempts to quit.

If you smoke, do this breathing exercise. It will help motivate you to quit and help you with your cravings for cigarettes when you do. Here's how:

1. Sit with your back straight. Place the tip of your tongue against the ridge of tissue behind your upper front teeth, and keep it there throughout the exercise.
2. Exhale completely through your mouth, making a *whoosh* sound.
3. Close your mouth and inhale quietly through your nose to a silent count of four.
4. Hold your breath for a count of seven.
5. Exhale completely through your mouth, again making a *whoosh* sound, to a count of eight.

6. This is one breath. Now inhale again and repeat the cycle three more times.

Do this throughout the day, whenever you crave a smoke.

If you smoke, you should take antioxidant vitamins and minerals, which to some extent can reverse the changes in respiratory tissue caused by tobacco, and so help protect against lung cancer. Also, increase your intake of dietary sources of carotenes (carrots, sweet potatoes, yellow and orange squash and fruits, and leafy green vegetables).

Good luck, and please set a date for your next attempt to quit.

Smoking Pot While Pregnant?

Q:

Has there been any research that suggests the effects of marijuana use during pregnancy?

A:

In general, it is wise to avoid putting any drugs into your body during the first three months of pregnancy, when most fetal development is taking place. It makes sense to take as few drugs as possible during the rest of the pregnancy as well.

Of the common recreational drugs in use, however, marijuana is probably less risky than nicotine, alcohol, and even caffeine. Coffee, for example, may increase the risk of miscarriage. Alcohol increases the probability of birth defects. Mothers who smoke cigarettes have more miscarriages and often give birth to babies with below-normal birth weights.

Marijuana is a less powerful pharmacological agent, so the adverse effects are likely to be less severe, although there is little evidence documenting them. One study reported in the *New England Journal of Medicine* in 1989 did associate marijuana use with impaired fetal growth.

The bottom line: Don't put foreign substances into your body during pregnancy, especially during the first trimester. Smoking (marijuana or cigarettes) around the baby is also not a good idea, since babies are very sensitive to smoke of all kinds.

Cut Out
That Snore?

Q:
*Outside of a drastic operation, what can I do to re-
duce or eliminate snoring?*

A:
Snoring results when the soft tissue of the airway relaxes and vibrates during sleep (this also may happen
when your nose is obstructed while you try to breathe).
It can range in severity from a bothersome nuisance to
real difficulty getting oxygen during the night. So far,
the loudest recorded snore has been 88 decibels, potentially enough to cause hearing loss with prolonged
exposure. Snoring is three times more common in
obese people, and its frequency increases with age.
I've seen a variety of estimates, but many agree that
about 60 percent of men and 40 percent of women
snore. Snoring tends to occur more often when people
sleep on their backs, because of the position of the airway structures.

There are several devices that are claimed to help
snorers. One is a battery-operated wristband called
the Mini Snore Control, from The Sharper Image,
that's activated by sound. Their toll-free number is
800 344-4444. When you start snoring, the device be-
gins to vibrate and wakes you enough so you can roll
over on your side. Usually that's enough to stop the
snore.

Another device fits on the nose and keeps the nasal passages open. It looks fairly easy to use and the manufacturer claims it dramatically reduces snoring. There are also pillows that keep the head and neck in a better position to avoid snoring. But I'm less enthusiastic about those.

What else can you do? Avoid alcoholic beverages, tranquilizers, sleeping pills, or antihistamines before going to bed. Try to sleep on your side or your stomach. Also, consider the possibility that you may have a nasal infection or allergy that is clogging your nose.

There is an operation to end snoring, as you say. Surgeons cut the uvula, the little organ that hangs down in the back of the throat, and get success in two-thirds of cases. But this surgery is painful and should only be used as a last resort.

I also recommend telling your sleeping partner that it's fine for him or her to wake you, roll you, or do whatever's necessary—other than asphyxiate you—to get you to stop. Pleasant dreams.

Additive-Free Sports Drinks?

Q:
Do you know of any energy drinks that are a bit lighter on the chemicals and better for you than Gatorade and the like? I am a runner and I enjoy these drinks but wonder if there isn't something out there that is better for me.

A:
I don't usually recommend commercial energy drinks, because they contain artificial dyes and other unhealthy additives.

When you exercise, you lose a lot of fluids and some minerals from exertion. Fluid loss can be major, especially if you're running in a hot climate or for longer than an hour. And dehydration can drastically impair performance and mental sharpness.

Energy drinks help most because they contain water, simple sugars, and electrolytes such as sodium and potassium. There's also evidence that drinking one of these before exercising may boost your ability to work out harder and longer, as long as you're doing something that doesn't require a lot of stops and starts. These drinks bring your blood sugar up to its normal operating range as you start to work out; while you're exercising, hormonal changes keep it steady. (If you stop or slow down significantly, your blood sugar may spike, and then fall when you start your workout again.) A caution: Don't use these drinks more than a few minutes before exercising, or you may feel a sharp drop in blood sugar once you start.

Whatever you do, drink lots of water. Drink more than you think you need. Studies have shown that recreational runners tend to drink less than they need—before, during, and after exercise. If you've lost a lot of salt or potassium from exercise, you can replace those substances by eating some fruits or vegetables. I don't know that there's a need for any kind of sports drink after exercise. But if you enjoy such drinks, look for natural versions that don't have additives and artificial colors. Health food stores carry them. Or you can make your own:

Natural Sports Drink

Over medium heat, dissolve 1/4 cup sugar in 2 cups of water. Add 1/4 tsp salt. Remove from stove, cool, and add 1/4 cup of orange juice. Mix with water to fill a quart bottle—and go!

Ouch! Relief for a Sprain?

Q:
I sprained my ankle four weeks ago. The swelling shrank considerably at first, but has remained on a plateau for the past three weeks and does not appear to be getting any better. What can I do for it? Do bad sprains normally take a long time to heal?

A:
The swelling of sprains should go down fairly quickly. If it doesn't, there may be some reason why the fluid is obstructed.

I have two suggestions. First, try acupuncture treatment. I have found acupuncture to work very effectively, especially for swollen knees; it reduces pain and speeds healing.

Second, take supplements of bromelain; you can buy it in capsules from health food stores. This is a pineapple enzyme that's used by some sports doctors. I've seen it dramatically reduce swelling from injuries. The dose is 200 to 400 milligrams, three times a day. Take it between meals, on an empty stomach—at least ninety minutes before or three hours after eating. (Some people are allergic to bromelain, so stop using it if you develop any itching.)

The best way to reduce swelling and blood flow during the first twenty-four hours after a sprain is to put ice on it right away. You can buy wraparound ice packs or just use a bag of frozen peas or some ice cubes in a towel. Try to keep the ice on as much as possible for the first few hours; after that, intermittent applications may be helpful. After twenty-four hours, you can start alternating heat and cold. Protect the sprain from further injury by using a wraparound bandage.

Either tincture of arnica or DMSO (dimethyl sulfoxide) may ease the pain and swelling. Arnica is a plant native to the high mountains of western North America that can be crushed whole and soaked in alcohol to produce a soothing liniment. Rub it in gently, but not into broken skin. Never ingest tincture of arnica; it's toxic. But you can take homeopathic arnica tablets in the 30x potency. Start with four tablets as soon as possible after the injury, then take four more every hour for the first day. Place the tablets under your tongue and let them dissolve. The next day, take four tablets every two hours. Then, the following day, cut back to four tablets four times a day. You may continue this for four or five days.

DMSO is a chemical made from wood pulp. It penetrates the skin and promotes healing. Paint a 70 percent solution of DMSO on the sore area with cotton and let it dry. You may feel warmth or stinging, and experience a garlicky taste in your mouth. Try it three times a day for three days. If there is no improvement, stop using it. If you do feel some improvement, apply DMSO twice a day for three more days, then once a day for a final three days.

Are Steroids Okay?

Q:
What's your opinion of steroids and protein drinks to enhance athletic performance?

A:
I'm opposed to the use of both kinds of products.

Anabolic steroids are sex hormones, usually synthetic, that increase protein metabolism, bone density, and muscle bulk. For some time, male athletes and bodybuilders have been taking anabolic steroids to build muscles and enhance performance. In fact, this practice is astonishingly common. Five years ago, the Drug Enforcement Administration made anabolic steroids controlled substances, ending legal prescription of them, but other sources have appeared. The promise of rapid development of big muscles and a powerful body image is very seductive, especially to teens and young men.

A study published July 4, 1996, in the *New England Journal of Medicine* reported that injections of testosterone (a natural anabolic steroid) added extra muscle and strength in a group of 40 male bodybuilders. *The New York Times* headline put it succinctly: TESTOSTERONE = BIG MUSCLES. That's not news, really. What's important to ask is: What's the downside?

There's plenty to talk about. It is widely accepted that steroids can have very significant adverse effects, including loss of sexual potency and drive and erratic mood swings. They also increase your risk of heart disease and high blood pressure and can cause acne, baldness, and abnormal liver function. Women may experience masculinizing changes, such as a deepened voice and increased facial hair. In fact, women were excluded from the recent study, because the potential side effects for them were considered unacceptable.

Proponents of steroids say these effects are rare. They will be encouraged by the *New England Journal of Medicine* study, which also found no evidence that steroids made the weight lifters more aggressive. I think it's important to note that the study was of short duration (ten weeks) and the dose of testosterone given was much lower than what most bodybuilders take.

In my view, steroids unbalance the body's hormonal system and ultimately lead to weakening of the body. High doses may be addictive.

As for protein supplements, I can see no reason to use them. I've seen competitive bodybuilders who developed liver dysfunction as a result of force-feeding on protein. Excess consumption of protein—in any form—puts an added workload on the digestive system, liver, and kidneys. Protein is not a very efficient fuel for the body. It takes more energy to digest and metabolize, and it breaks down into toxic residues that the liver and kidneys must handle. The breakdown products of protein metabolism can also irritate the immune system.

Cramped by Stitches?

Q:
When running, I get what often is referred to as a stitch—a pain in the abdominal area just below the rib cage. What causes this? What can I do for it?

A:
The pain you're feeling is probably a spasm of one of the muscles in the abdominal wall or between the ribs. The cause could be any one of many possibilities. Perhaps you're running in a way that puts an unequal strain on a particular muscle. You may be more fatigued than you realize. Or you may be depleted in sodium or potassium from exertion. Cramps like this aren't very well understood, but it's believed they involve depletion of muscle nutrients, fluid loss, and electrolyte imbalance.

Stretching more before running probably won't make any difference. Even the best-conditioned athletes get stitches unpredictably. Interestingly (and ironically), people who do not exercise regularly and are in poor condition are less likely to get them.

I'll admit stitches can really hurt, but I don't think the abdominal pain you're experiencing is anything to be concerned about. It can be so strong, though, that you lose your balance and fall. Maybe it's just a sign that you should stop your run right then and rest a little bit.

To ease the pain, gently stretch the muscle. If you've made it home and you still hurt, apply an ice pack to relax the muscle and reduce swelling.

If you want to provide your muscles with more energy, herbs can help your body process carbohydrates and absorb oxygen more efficiently. They also can boost muscle recovery after exercise. You can try licorice, ginseng, or schizandra berries to boost your muscles' stamina. Kathi Keville offers a recipe incorporating all of them in *Herbs for Health and Healing:*

> 1 teaspoon tincture of Siberian ginseng root
> 1/2 teaspoon each tinctures of shizandra berries, ginseng root, saw palmetto berries, and licorice root
>
> Combine ingredients. Take 1/2 dropperful twice a day, or as needed for stamina.

Why the Stye?

Q:
I have been getting styes lately. Would you know what causes them? Is it a bacterial infection or lack of a nutrient?

A:
Styes are bacterial infections of the tear duct. The technical name is hordeolum, usually caused by staph. They can be quite painful and disfiguring, causing the area around the eye to redden and swell. Usually they go away on their own, with patience.

Styes on the outside of your eyelid eventually will rupture, discharge pus, then disappear. Inside your eyelid, the infection can be more severe. You can speed the resolution of the problem by applying hot compresses for ten minutes a couple of times a day. Topical antibiotics usually don't help much.

Recurrence is not unusual. But if you're getting these regularly it would be a good idea to look for an underlying cause, such as contact lenses or exposure to cigarette smoke. Styes are contagious and can be transmitted by finger contact. But most people don't get them because the immune system protects the eyes pretty well. Our tears contain antibodies that eliminate bacteria before they get a chance to settle in. Sometimes the appearance of a stye can indicate a temporary depression of immunity.

I don't know of any nutritional lack that would cause styes, but it might be worth trying a regimen of vitamin C. I'd suggest 3,000 to 6,000 milligrams of vitamin C a day, in three equal doses, to see if this reduces the frequency of the infections you're experiencing.

Blocking Sunburn Damage?

Q:
After shaving my head I spent a weekend in the Rocky Mountain sun. Despite putting on an SPF-30 sunscreen, I woke up Monday morning with a blistering, crusty, pus-spewing top. Now it's better and the skin is just peeling, but do I have anything to be concerned about?

A:
Ouch.

The incidence of skin cancer is rising at an alarming rate, with ultraviolet (UV) radiation from the sun the major cause. One reason may be the weakening of the Earth's protective ozone layer as a result of atmospheric pollution, so that more solar radiation is now reaching us. Even though UV waves are longer and have less energy than ionizing radiation like X rays, they are still powerful enough to penetrate living cells in the skin and cause DNA damage. UV radiation doesn't just hurt the skin; it can also cause loss of vision as you grow older by damaging the retina (macular degeneration) and the lens (cataract).

I always recommend protecting yourself in as many ways as possible. Stay out of the sun when it's at a high angle in the sky. Choose clothing that covers your skin—brimmed hats, light-weight, long-sleeve shirts. Use a powerful sunscreen (SPF-15, at least) that blocks both UVA and UVB, and wear UV-protective sunglasses. And, finally, take anti-oxidants to help block the chemical reactions that can lead to cancer. Living in the Arizona desert, I try to follow this advice year-round.

Cancer risks increase with cumulative exposure, so you should definitely avoid getting another burn on your head. The more bad burns you get, especially in your teenage years and in your twenties, the higher your risk of skin cancer as you age. If you stop getting burned, you will lessen the danger.

Most dermatologists say it's a good idea to get in the habit of putting a high-SPF sunscreen on every morning. I agree. But as you've found, sunscreen can give you a false sense of protection. Just because you're wearing sunscreen, don't assume you can spend unlimited time in the sun. It's still good to be careful. You got in trouble because you were at a high altitude, where thinner atmosphere lets more UV radiation in. You needed even more protection than your sunscreen gave you.

An old-fashioned sunscreen that is still effective is zinc oxide. This is an opaque cream that provides a mechanical barrier to sunlight. (It's now available in neon colors as well as in the original white.) It works extremely well if you don't mind walking around with your face completely white or electric blue.

If you do get burned, aloe is probably the most soothing treatment. You can buy bottles of the pure gel in health food stores or grow the plants around your house.

Need to Dry Out Swimmer's Ear?

Q:
What's the best medicine for swimmer's ear?

A:
The best way to treat "swimmer's ear," like just about anything, is to avoid getting it in the first place (use wax or silicone earplugs). But if it's too late for that, make a mixture of equal parts white vinegar and rubbing alcohol. Get in the habit of rinsing your ears out with this potion when you come out of a pool or the ocean. Then gently dry your ears with a cotton swab.

Other preventive measures include shaking your head when you get out of the pool to expel trapped water. You can also place the tip of some clean facial tissue, twisted into a point, into each ear for about ten seconds to soak up the moisture. Don't remove earwax from your ears (unless it's a problem), because it helps protect the ear canal.

Once you've got swimmer's ear, you're probably going to have to treat it with an antibiotic solution like Neosporin, which comes in a form specifically for ears.

I have two favorite remedies for earaches: garlic oil and mullein oil. Warm either of these oils slightly, then use a dropper to put a few drops in the ear that is hurting. Plug it loosely with cotton. To make garlic oil, crush a few cloves into some olive oil and let it sit for a few days, then strain it. Some people put a small piece of peeled raw garlic directly into the ear—it eventually dissolves. You can find mullein oil in health food stores. It's made by steeping the flowers from mullein—*Verbascum thapsus,* a common roadside weed—in olive oil. Apply it the same way as the garlic oil. Try it, it really works.

Burning for a Quick Tan?

Q:
How bad is it to self-tan? Is it any better for you than the sun?

A:
People can't seem to get away from the idea that a tan is healthy and beautiful. That's why there are self-tanning lotions and tanning salons.

The lotions are harmless, but the results never quite look natural to me. Fortunately, there are now improved formulas that at least don't leave you streaked with orange. The new products contain dehydroxyacetone, which interacts with proteins in the surface cells of your skin. Some people complain about a slight chemical or metallic scent, but that goes away in a few hours.

To avoid blotches, you need to be careful when applying the lotion. First, get rid of dry, flaky skin with a sponge or washcloth. Remove your rings and other jewelry, and apply the tanner lightly just as you would a body lotion. Put only a little on your knees and elbows—the dry skin will absorb more color than the rest of your body. Try not to get the lotion under your nails, since it will discolor them, and wash your hands immediately so your palms don't look unnaturally tan. Then, remember that even though your skin is more brown, it's not protected by the melanin produced by a natural suntan. So be sure to use lots of sunscreen before going out in the sun. Apply the sunscreen only after the tanning lotion is completely dry.

As for tanning salons, my advice is to stay away. The rays in a tanning parlor can actually be stronger than ordinary sunshine. A study in Sweden a couple of years ago found that people under age thirty who used tanning salons more than ten times a year had a seven-times-higher risk of melanoma than other people. Most skin cancer is related to UV radiation, and melanoma is the deadliest kind. There's no such thing as "tanning" rays, as distinct from "burning" rays. The UV-A light of tanning salons is at least as harmful as the UV-B rays you get during peak sunlight hours.

Sometimes people go to tanning salons before they go on a winter vacation in order to avoid a sunburn. A better technique is to expose yourself gradually to the sun once you've arrived, and be sure to use a sunblock of at least SPF-15.

I'm not one of those doctors who would have you avoid sun at any cost, but a tan is definitely not a sign of health. The only good thing about a suntan is that it means you've been outdoors, where you may have been getting exercise, relaxing, and having fun. To get tan in a shop, without the associated healthful activities, is not quite what the doctor ordered.

How's Now
with the Tao?

Q:
What are your impressions of the Chinese Tao of sex? Claims are that by withholding ejaculation the body is strengthened, the mind made clearer, vision and hearing are improved, and the man feels closer to and more loving toward his mate. As reluctant as I may be to accept the concept completely, my limited experience with the Taoist approach seems to indicate more truth than fiction. Any comments?

A:
It is a widespread folk belief, especially in east Asia, that withholding semen improves mental and physical health. In ancient Chinese sexology, reserving semen was believed to prolong life and maybe lead to immortality. Something of the same belief is part of the mythology of modern sports, too. ("Don't have sex before the big game.") I don't know that there's any evidence to support the idea that infrequent ejaculation preserves health, however, or if anyone has ever done research to find out.

In thinking about the Tao of love, I think it's best not to become preoccupied with ejaculation. Over the years, the ancient Chinese theories about sex have become distorted to the point where they make sex seem like a war between men and women, in which men may seriously harm themselves by sacrificing their semen. Semen becomes a symbol of male power and life force that females covet, like vampires who suck the blood of their prey.

That's not what the Tao of love should be about. If a man can let go of the desire to ejaculate, he can relax and enjoy the peaks and valleys of lovemaking longer. Instead of thinking in terms of reaching a goal, he can concentrate on the ecstasy of touching his lover, and his lover's responses. There is time to savor each other's texture, scent, and movements.

For a woman, it's the same. Instead of striving toward orgasm, she can enjoy the pleasures of touching, caressing, and kissing. The techniques of Taoist sex reflect one underlying purpose: Rather than letting sexual energy control us, men and women should learn to control it with conscious intent. Since an ejaculation necessitates a temporary end to lovemaking, if a man can learn to enjoy the experience in other ways, the night can be very long, and very pleasurable.

For an understanding of the Taoist philosophy, I recommend two books by Jolan Chang: *The Tao of Love and Sex* and *The Tao of the Loving Couple*.

Will the Ringing Ever Stop?

Q:

I'm a massage therapist. One of my clients has experienced ringing in his ears for months. The only treatment his doctors advise is to continue on steroids, even though there has not been noticeable improvement. I read in Spontaneous Healing *about a German physician who experienced great success with yoga and stress relief techniques. Can you recommend an alternative? Any herbs?*

A:

Tinnitus—ringing in the ears—was relatively rare when I was in medical school, but it's definitely not rare these days. It has become almost epidemic in the United States, and there's not really any clear understanding among medical doctors of its cause. It seems to affect people of all ages, and the medical treatments for it aren't very good. Some people think it's due to a viral infection, but that's just the ready Western answer to many medical riddles.

What you hear are noises that come from inside the body and won't go away. It feels as if there's no way to escape, which can be most annoying. The noises can make it hard to hear other people's voices, to concentrate, or to sleep through the night.

As I wrote in *Spontaneous Healing,* my German physician friend, Helmut Milz, M.D., of Marquartstein,

Bavaria, works at a psychosomatic medical clinic and regards tinnitus as a stress-related condition. He believes that chronic muscle tension in the head and neck interferes with blood circulation to the inner ear. If he's right, then increased use of computers, television watching, and the general stress in our culture could explain why there is so much more tinnitus these days.

I would recommend two approaches. First, your client should do some kind of stress reduction technique aimed specifically at improving posture and relaxing muscles. I would recommend yoga, or bodywork such as the Alexander technique. I would also suggest acupuncture.

Second, I would use the herb ginkgo (*Ginkgo biloba*). Ginkgo is nontoxic and increases blood circulation in the head and neck. Many people report improvement with it. Your client would need to take it for at least two months before making a decision about its usefulness. The dose is two tablets of the standardized extract three times a day, with meals.

Check out Richard Hallam's book *Tinnitus: Dealing with the Ringing in Your Ears,* which is based on the philosophy that the best way to deal with ringing is to stop fighting it. Hallam, who is a psychologist, helps readers learn to tolerate the sounds until they stop being annoying and aren't particularly noticeable. Another good resource is the American Tinnitus Association in Portland, Oregon.

Is My Toothbrush Alive?

Q:
I'm concerned about bacteria or whatever growing on my toothbrush. How often would you advise changing to a new toothbrush? Is it advisable to disinfect a toothbrush between uses, perhaps by soaking it in salt solution?

A:
First of all, never exchange toothbrushes with another person. That's an easy way to spread colds and other infections. In particular, it's possible to contract hepatitis B, C, or D if you share a toothbrush with someone who's already infected. Virus-infected blood and bodily fluids are the known modes of transmission. HIV can also be transmitted by sharing personal items like toothbrushes and razors (through infected blood, not saliva). Bottom line: It's always better to spend the extra buck or two and get a new toothbrush rather than share. Keep an extra in your medicine cabinet.

With your own toothbrush, bacteria won't be that much of a problem if you use a toothpaste with an antibacterial agent like tea tree oil (from the leaves of *Melaleuca alternifolia*) or chlorine dioxide in it. Just go ahead and air dry the brush in a place that's fairly sanitary—away from the toilet, for example, and not in the trajectory of splashes from the sink.

It's good to change toothbrushes fairly frequently—

say, every two or three months. This will keep your brushing effective, in addition to keeping your tooth-brush cleaner.

While we're on the subject, here are some brushing basics: Use a brush with soft bristles, so you don't damage your teeth or gums. Brush gently at least twice a day, holding your toothbrush at a 45-degree angle. Use small circular motions. Scrubbing your tongue will get rid of bacteria and freshen your breath. Remember: To avoid damaging your gums, don't brush too hard.

Electric toothbrushes sound great but I've never grown to like any of them. Some dentists love the ultra-sonic ones that emit inaudible high-frequency sound waves to kill bacteria while you're brushing. Use these appliances if you want, but a plain old manual toothbrush does the job just fine.

Don't forget to floss!

What the $#@%!?

Q:
Tourette's syndrome is a disorder hallmarked by involuntary motor and vocal tics. Any info on new findings about this disorder? Any suggestions on natural therapies to relieve the symptoms? Some say it is related to obsessive-compulsive disorder. Any thoughts on this?

A:
Since Tourette's syndrome has become better known, many people are delighted by the concept—especially the thought of being able to yell "fuck" in public and get away with it.

But, of course, it's not that simple. As you say, people who have the disease experience a variety of uncontrollable "tics" that can range from simple motions like blinking to complex activities like bending over and touching the ground. People may also grunt, clear their throats, or bark. Inappropriate swearing, making obscene gestures, and compulsive imitation of others can also occur in this neuropsychiatric disorder, but they are far less common. More common, and very disturbing to Touretters, are surges of uncontrollable rage and other strong emotions.

A French neurologist named Georges Gille de la Tourette first identified the syndrome in 1885 after observing several patients, including a French noblewoman, the Marquise de Dampierre, who would make sudden bizarre cries in the middle of polite conversation. Until a couple of decades ago it was considered a psychiatric disorder, mostly of boys, brought on by poor parenting skills.

Now there's considerable evidence for a genetic root, combined with prenatal environmental factors and birth complications. Children with Tourette's often were exposed before birth to high levels of tobacco smoke, coffee, or alcohol. It's estimated that more than 100,000 Americans have the syndrome, with only one out of every four male. The syndrome is less associated with uninhibited angry outbursts in women, so some people speculate that the quiet, odd actions of young girls and women with the condition often go unnoticed and undiagnosed.

There are strong links with obsessive-compulsive disorder (OCD)—and a number of other psychiatric problems. Touretters often show obsessive-compulsive behavior like washing their hands repeatedly, as well as attention-deficit hyperactivity disorder (ADHD), and anxiety.

In fact, these symptoms often cause far more distress to the person than does Tourette's syndrome itself. And they can be difficult to treat, because the stimulants given for ADHD, for example, tend to worsen the tics. But many Touretters don't take any medication at all. As they grow older, they become practiced and comfortable explaining their condition to others when the tics happen in public. And they learn to suppress them. Family counseling and therapy are good ways to help the whole family deal with the stigma of socially unacceptable—or at least unusual—behavior.

The tics get worse under stress, so there's an obvious place to begin to find natural solutions to the problem. Biofeedback, relaxation techniques, and exercise may help. And some people have used the surges of behavioral changes as a creative resource. In his book *The Man Who Mistook His Wife for a Hat,* Oliver Sacks writes about a surgeon with Tourette's who maintains an active practice and skillfully performs extremely complex operations. Some people think Mozart had Tourette's.

To learn more about the disease, I suggest reading *A Mind of Its Own: Tourette's Syndrome, A Story and a Guide,* by Ruth Dowling Bruun and Bertel Bruun. There's also a film, *Twitch and Shout,* by Laurel Chiton, which you can get through New Day Films in New Jersey. Other resources include the Tourette Syndrome Association in Bayside, New York.

Help for
Tummy Trouble?

Q:

People like me with stomach complaints such as heart-burn, abdominal bloating, or gas pains are generously prescribed drugs such as Pepcid, Zantac, Tagamet, or Prilosec. Most of these drugs have potential long-term side effects, usually underplayed by Western doctors. Could you recommend gentler, natural remedies for these problems? Also, what lifestyle changes may help?

A:

Digestive disorders often can be traced to poor eating habits and stress. The gastrointestinal tract is very susceptible to the disturbing influence of stress, because it relies on complex coordination by the autonomic nervous system.

The licorice extract DGL (deglycyrrhizinated licorice) is an excellent natural remedy for all the problems you mention. DGL increases the mucous coating of the stomach, making it more resistant to the effects of acid. It is nontoxic and inexpensive, and it works better than prescription drugs. The prescription drugs act by suppressing acid production in the stomach. The problem with this approach is that you're not really getting to the root problem. As soon as you stop taking these drugs, there's going to be a rebound production of acid. If you deal with the problem by using DGL, you increase the body's defensive strength.

DGL is available as tablets or powder. Chew one to two tablets or take ¼ teaspoon of the powder fifteen minutes before meals and again at bedtime. Allow the material to dissolve slowly in your mouth and run down your throat.

For stomach problems generally, a number of herbal remedies can help. Peppermint tea is wonderful for nausea, indigestion, and some cases of heartburn (but because it relaxes the sphincter where the esophagus joins the stomach, it can worsen esophageal reflux syndrome, in which stomach acid irritates the lower esophagus). In general, it soothes the lining of the digestive tract. Buy pure peppermint tea, brew it in a covered container to retain the volatile components, and drink it hot or iced. Chamomile is also excellent for heartburn and indigestion, and will not aggravate esophageal reflux. You can buy it in tea bags in the supermarket. Steep in hot water in a covered container for ten minutes, and then enjoy.

I also feel strongly that people with stomach problems should not rely solely on remedies. Try looking for the causes of your problems, which probably have to do with excess consumption of stomach irritants like coffee, other forms of caffeine, decaffeinated coffee, alcohol, and foods (or food combinations) that you don't tolerate well. Smoking is another cause of stomach distress. I'd encourage you to make some dietary experiments to see if you can reduce symptoms and thereby eliminate the problem. A simple rule: Pay attention to—and stop eating—what makes your stomach hurt. Try eating smaller amounts more frequently. And work on reducing stress in your life.

Does Transcendental Meditation Work?

Q:

Transcendental meditation (TM) proponents maintain that the technique has far-reaching stress-reduction benefits, even going as far as to say it "can reverse the signs of aging" if practiced correctly. Are you familiar with any medical studies that have attempted to confirm the claims of TM enthusiasts?

A:

Transcendental meditation (TM) first became popular in the United States in the 1960s when the Beatles, Mia Farrow, the Beach Boys, and other celebrities took it up. The practice, based on ancient yogic teachings, applies a simple meditation technique that involves the repetition of a Sanskrit word or phrase—called a mantra—to prevent distracting thoughts. The four key elements to eliciting a relaxation response are a quiet environment, an object to dwell upon (like a word or symbol), a comfortable position, and, most important, a passive attitude that allows thoughts, images, and feelings to drift into your awareness and pass on through. Meditation is a way to break addiction to thought—to place your attention in present reality.

Proponents of TM have made some extreme claims that their method will reverse the effects of aging, allow people to levitate, and cause them to reach enlightenment. I'm sorry to say I haven't seen evidence for any of this, and you're wise to question them. But here's the good news. Studies on TM at Harvard Medical School in the mid-seventies showed it to lower oxygen consumption, increase blood flow, and slow heart rate, leading to a deep relaxation. Researchers also found TM to lower levels of blood lactate, which is associated with anxiety, and to decrease blood pressure in people with hypertension. You might look at Herbert Benson's book *The Relaxation Response,* which offers an excellent overview of this research.

I believe that other forms of meditation offer similar benefits, and, unlike TM, many are free. I don't recommend meditation for everyone; some people aren't ready for it, and some need simpler techniques for relaxing.

Cranberries for Urinary Tract Infections?

Q:

What is the latest on cranberries and urinary tract infections? If cranberries do help, can one use cranberry supplements rather than juice for the same effect?

A:

Urinary tract infections occur when bacteria such as *E. coli*, which normally live in the bowel, make their way into the bladder and set up residence. Cranberry juice, long recommended as a folk remedy for the problem, has held up under scientific scrutiny. In a study published in the *Journal of the American Medical Association,* women who drank cranberry juice were 58 percent less likely to develop a urinary tract infection than those who drank a placebo (another red drink containing vitamin C). If they already had an infection, they were 27 percent less likely to have their infections continue if they drank cranberry juice. Advocates of cranberry juice treatment used to think it worked by acidifying the urine, making it less hospitable to bacteria. But now it appears that cranberries (and blueberries) contain a substance that disrupts the glue that bacteria use to adhere to tissue, making it harder for them to get established on the lining of the bladder.

I'm with you on skipping the juice. Cranberry

juice—at least the ordinary variety—is full of sugar and water, with only some of the real stuff. The high sugar content may actually encourage the growth of bacteria and yeast.

So my preference is to drink unsweetened cranberry juice concentrate, which you can buy in a health food store, or to buy capsules of cranberry extract. The Eclectic Institute makes a freeze-dried product that's good. Take two capsules twice a day. Even if you're taking pharmaceutical drugs to treat the infection, I'd still take cranberry along with them.

Another herbal treatment for bladder infections is uva ursi, also known as bearberry (*Arctostaphylos uva-ursi*). This kills bacteria and reduces inflammation. But don't use it for more than a week, because it can irritate your kidneys and upset your stomach. Also, you must keep your urine alkaline in order for the uva ursi to work. That means eating lots of fruits and vegetables, especially potatoes. For a little extra antibacterial punch, eat garlic, nasturtium, parsley, and rose hips whenever you can.

You can also take some measures to help prevent a return of the infection. Avoid tight pants, synthetic underwear, and deodorant soaps, all of which can encourage bacteria. Also, many women get urinary tract infections shortly after a pelvic exam. Drinking a glass of water just before and after visiting your gynecologist seems to help protect against this problem.

Is Urine the Water of Life?

Q:

Not long ago, Yoga Journal *had an article on urine therapy. This is quite a bugaboo for those of us in the West. The article referred to a book,* Your Own Perfect Medicine, *which really sang the praises of pee! Do you have any experience with this treatment, and if so, what is your opinion of it?*

A:

Urine therapy refers to the drinking of one's own urine for therapeutic benefit. This unusual practice originated in India. Occasionally, I come across folk remedies in our culture involving topical applications of urine, which I have no problem with. Enough people report good effects with it in conditions like athlete's foot and jellyfish stings to make me think it works, and I am not upset at the thought of having urine on the skin.

But the drinking of urine is a different matter. Some proponents of urine therapy say you can rid yourself of herpes, AIDS, and leprosy by drinking your own urine. Not long ago, about 600 proponents gathered in India for three days to compare notes on the practice, which they claimed could reverse conditions ranging from arthritis to cancer. Those who recommend urine therapy point to the complexity of the fluid and relate its components to the life-giving properties of blood.

When I think about drinking urine, I find myself up against a major psychological barrier. There are two parts to this: a gut-level revulsion and an intellectual conviction that urine drinking violates a clear intent of the body to rid itself of waste. As a practitioner of natural medicine, I find it hard to get past the idea that the body wants to get rid of urine. Urine does contain hormones and other bioactive substances that might produce therapeutic effects. But my impression is that the benefits being reported are placebo responses activated by confronting and breaking a powerful psychological taboo. I would not stand in the way of anyone who wanted to try urine therapy, but for myself and my family, I prefer to seek out treatments that are more to my taste.

Walking for Your Life?

Q:
Is it true that walking is almost equal to jogging as an aerobic exercise?

A:
I'm a great proponent of walking. Not only is it almost equal to jogging in terms of getting your heart pumping, but I think research eventually will show that it's superior in terms of overall health benefits. There are many reasons to prefer walking to just about any other form of exercise. First of all, everyone knows how to do it and it doesn't require any equipment. Second, you can do it anywhere. Third, the risk of injury is far less than for any other kind of aerobic exercise.

With running, the risk of injury is high. Runners who go for endorphin highs often run through warning pain—then wind up being unable to exercise at all. They may also become exercise addicts.

I sometimes take a morning walk after I meditate. Or in the afternoon, I might walk around the ranch where I live. If I'm in a city like New York or San Francisco, I try to do as much walking as possible. San Francisco is great because of the hills, and in New York the people-watching always keeps me entertained.

You may find walking meditative and relaxing. As you do it, you can take in the sights or listen to something on a Walkman. Walking exercises your brain as well as your body; its cross-patterned movement (right arm moves forward with the left leg) generates harmonizing electrical activity in your brain.

I find that good running shoes with cushioned soles are best for walking. But experiment—find out what works for you. If you walk up a long, gradual hill or walk at a good clip, you can get your heart and respiratory rates high enough to produce the aerobic conditioning you need. Maintain good posture and be sure to swing your arms as you go. I recommend forty-five minutes of walking a day. That's about three miles. Do it at least five times a week.

What's the Best Water Filter?

Q:

I know there are a lot of contaminants and toxins in water these days. What do you recommend for a water filter?

A:

Water quality varies from place to place, so you should have your water tested to see what impurities it contains. The results will help you decide whether you actually need a filter and what type to get. Note that it can cost more than $100 to test for a range of contaminants.

Chlorine and lead are the two most common problems. Chlorine is a powerful oxidizing agent that can cause birth defects, cancer, and heart disease. As for lead, even very small amounts can be harmful, especially to young children. Lead poisoning causes organ damage and stunts the nervous system, producing mental retardation.

In many cities, public health officials are also finding *Cryptosporidium* in water; this is a microbe that can cause great harm to people with compromised immune systems.

Check out the different kinds of filtration systems available, making sure to find out how often you need to change filters, how much the replacements cost, and how difficult they are to install. Systems vary in quality, efficiency, and price.

Six systems are available for purifying water at home. None of them is perfect. Each has distinct strengths and drawbacks. Always read the labeling to learn exactly what the product claims to remove.

Steam distillation is the surest method. Water is heated to boiling, the steam collected and cooled until it condenses again without the impurities. This method works, but it's the most expensive one. Distillation will not remove a few volatile organic compounds, which boil over with the steam.

Carbon filtration is probably the most popular system. Units containing specially prepared, porous carbon attach under the sink or at the tap. Carbon filtration is good for removing chlorine, toxic organic molecules, and bad tastes from water, but it doesn't capture heavy metals or minerals. The system is fast, but it stops working as soon as the carbon becomes saturated with contaminants. Also, as the carbon collects organic matter, it becomes a breeding ground for bacteria. Bacteria will pour out into your first glass of water of the day, unless you take a minute to flush the filter first.

Ion exchange rids water of dissolved minerals and toxic metals, but it is less efficient at removing organic molecules. It works through charged particles in the filter that exchange themselves for charged particles in the water. These filters normally employ sodium in the exchange, so unless there's another process to remove it later, you could end up with harmful levels of sodium in the purified water. Water purified by this method will corrode pipes, carrying metals out of them. I don't recommend it.

Purifiers that use ultraviolet light to kill micro-organisms have no effect on chemical contaminants.

In the past, I used a system called reverse osmosis (RO). RO removes minerals and toxic metals like lead, along with organic contaminants (and *Cryptosporidium*). In an RO unit, water pressure forces water through an osmotic membrane (one with tiny holes that allow small water molecules, but not contaminant molecules, to pass through). Bacteria are blocked, and they don't grow on the filter. This may be the best way to go. However, you should know that the process is slow, and wastes a lot of water, which is why I finally stopped using it. I can't afford to waste water in the desert. RO water is also very corrosive to pipes, so place the system near the tap.

A newer system that looks good combines a solid carbon block filter with a copper-zinc alloy called KDF. This dual cartridge system removes most impurities and is affordable and simple. The KDF puts small amounts of copper and zinc into the water, which most experts consider healthful.

Energized by Wheatgrass?

Q:
What do you think of wheatgrass? I've heard that 1 ounce supposedly contains as much nutritional value as 2.5 pounds of vegetables. Is that true?

A:
Wheatgrass is a sprouted grain that grows naturally in pastures. Cattle love it—but only when it's nice and green. These days, you're likely to see gardens of wheatgrass in juice bars and health food stores, along with green powders and tablets. Wheatgrass enthusiasts use juice from the young shoots in all sorts of ways, from juice drinks to enemas. They use it as part of a regimen for treating cancer and for building up the body's immunity.

Wheatgrass is supposed to have high life energy and many other positive attributes. You'll find claims that it will clean your blood, repair your DNA, deodorize your body, keep your hair from turning gray, help your pet, confer energy, and lengthen your life. The chlorophyll is supposed to act as an antioxidant and the nutrients are thought to provide an energy lift.

Unfortunately, despite wheatgrass's wide popularity, there's no evidence to back any of these claims. And I don't recommend its use other than as a source of minerals and vitamins. If you like wheatgrass and it appeals to you, fine. Drink it. But I don't think it's a substitute for 2.5 pounds of vegetables. Besides, I don't like the way it tastes.

How to Beat the Winter Blues?

Q:

What have you heard about SAD (seasonal affective disorder)? Since I was diagnosed, I have been experimenting, and a few years ago reasoned that if feverfew affects serotonin uptake for migraines, it might work for SAD. It has been quite beneficial used in conjunction with full-spectrum lighting.

A:

Winter is the time of year when people with seasonal affective disorder start to feel bad. People who have it usually know it—but not always. It's a depression, often severe, that comes on in winter months and is believed to be related to lack of exposure to light. People feel lethargic, irritable, and depressed; many crave carbohydrates and tend to gain weight. It's more common in the northern latitudes, affecting many people in Alaska, for example, and few here in southern Arizona. Twice as many women as men experience this disorder.

There are two treatments recommended for SAD. First, exposure to a small amount of full-spectrum light has really helped some people. Even ordinary artificial light seems to work—at least thirty minutes a day at 10,000 lux (20 times normal indoor lighting). It may take three to four weeks to feel the full effect. It would also be a good idea to exercise outdoors in the middle of the day, looking up toward the sky (but not directly into the sun) now and then. The authority on light treatment for SAD is John Ott, who has written several books on the subject.

Many people also believe that abnormal levels of melatonin are related to SAD, because melatonin is involved in the body's reaction to light and dark, and affects brain function. Melatonin also helps set the body's internal clock. Some SAD patients have been found to have an unusual delay in their melatonin rhythms. Taking melatonin at night could help, but on the other hand it could make things worse. Melatonin secretion peaks around midnight. It normally increases in winter; in the summer months it drops in women and is unchanged in men.

I don't really know the consequences of taking melatonin on a long-term basis. But for short periods of time it's probably okay. I'd suggest no more than 1 milligram taken at bedtime.

You ask about feverfew (*Tenacetum parthenium*) and serotonin. I don't think the method by which feverfew works for migraine is known. And I don't think we know that feverfew affects serotonin uptake. But feverfew is harmless and would be interesting to try. I'd like to know the results. I'd get an extract of feverfew that is standardized for content of parthenolides. Take one tablet or capsule twice a day over a couple of months and see if you notice an effect.

There is a national support group for people with SAD. It's called the National Organization for SAD.

What's the Perfect Workout?

Q:
How many calories should you be burning during an average workout? I tend to do half an hour of cardio-vascular exercise three times a week, plus occasional weight training. According to the machines, I burn 250 calories. I'm five feet four and weigh 125 pounds. Is this the right amount of exercise and calorie-burning for me?

A:
Aerobic exercise is the kind that increases your heart rate and makes you huff and puff. It promotes general fitness, conditions your heart and respiratory system, and increases stamina. It also tones your nervous and immune systems, reduces stress, increases the flow of oxygen throughout the body, and gives you a sense of strength and well-being.

For optimum cardiovascular fitness, I recommend exercising every day. Aim toward at least thirty minutes five times a week. It need not be in one continuous session. Ideally, your daily routine should also include plenty of aerobic activity, such as brisk walking, housework, gardening, and so on.

I am a great proponent of walking for fitness. Sustained walking—especially uphill walking and brisk walking—can give a better overall workout than running or exercising intensely on aerobic machines. Walking has the advantages of not requiring any equipment and carrying the least risk of injury of any aerobic exercise. Use good posture, swing your arms, and keep a good pace. Three miles should take about forty-five minutes. I recommend running shoes for this activity—ones with well-cushioned insoles.

Specific forms of exercise have their own benefits. Swimming is great for the joints, a balanced muscular workout, and relaxation. Cycling builds knee muscles and can provide a feeling of exhilaration. Dancing is one of the best aerobic activities of all, because it's fun, never boring, and it provides a thorough workout.

Once you have developed good habits of regular exercise, you can add stretching, muscle toning, and strengthening to your routine. Yoga is a great way to stretch, improve flexibility, and experience deep relaxation. Breathing exercises, meditation, and other forms of relaxation are important to help neutralize stress.

Personally, I walk whenever possible. I use a Stair-Master occasionally, and go mountain biking in the desert. I also swim and do some weight training—and mix all of these up.

I don't think that calorie-burning is the best guide to how much exercise you should do. If your weight is stable, think in terms of overall cardiovascular fitness, strength, and flexibility. Vary your workout to keep it interesting. And, above all, have fun.

Yams for Hormone Therapy?

Q:
What's the scoop on wild yam cream? Is it merely a marketing phenomenon? Or does it have real botanical benefits for PMS sufferers and menopausal discomfort relief-seekers?

A:
Wild yam, or *Dioscorea,* is the tuber of a tropical plant. Don't expect to find it in your grocery store— it's completely unrelated to the sweet potatoes that many people call yams in this country. All sorts of claims have been made about wild yam because it contains a precursor of steroid hormones called diosgenin, which was used as the starting material for the first birth control pill. But diosgenin itself has no hormonal activity. Nor can the human body convert it into something that does.

That's why I question the efficacy of creams that contain only wild yam as the supposed source of natural hormonal activity. Some of these creams may contain a natural form of progesterone synthesized from diosgenin, even though this doesn't show up on the label. That would certainly make them active.

Wild yam may have sedative properties that can help relieve premenstrual problems. In *Herbs for Health and Healing,* Kathi Keville recommends a tea made of

1 teaspoon vitex berries, 1 teaspoon wild yam, $1/2$ teaspoon each of burdock root, dandelion root, feverfew leaves, and the flowering parts of hops. Place the herbs in a pot containing a quart of water and bring to a boil. Then steep for at least twenty minutes with the heat off. It may help with the cramps, emotional changes, and nausea you sometimes feel before your menstrual period. You can also buy a tincture with these herbs.

Natural Help for Yeast Infections?

Q:

What do I do about recurring yeast infections? I've had them for over twenty years.

A:

Many women suffer from frequent vaginal yeast infections, which can indicate an underlying metabolic imbalance. It often helps if you change your diet to make your body a less appealing host for the organism. Your partner may want to do the same. (Studies suggest that treating the patient's sexual partner may stop recurrence.)

First, try reducing your sugar intake. High-sugar diets stimulate the growth of yeast. Also, add garlic to your diet. A clove once a day is a powerful natural medicine, with specific anti-yeast effects. (That's one segment from a bulb, not the whole thing!) Mash or chop it fine, mix it with food, and eat it with a meal. Or cut it into chunks and swallow the chunks like pills. Fresh garlic is much better than any garlic supplement. Chew a little parsley afterward if you're concerned about odor—but if you eat garlic regularly and have a good attitude about it, you won't smell of it. Try it, it really works.

Finally, take acidophilus culture. These bacteria are the ones that make milk sour. "Friendly" and natural to the intestinal tract, they may also out-compete yeast in the vaginal area and change the chemistry of the tissues to make them resistant to the fungi. You can buy acidophilus in health food stores, in capsules or in a milk or carrot-juice base. Check the expiration date to make sure the bacteria are viable. Take 1 tablespoon of the liquid culture or one to two of the dry capsules after meals, unless the label directs otherwise.

These changes to your diet may help reverse some of your underlying susceptibility to yeast infections. To treat the infections when they occur, try placing a capsule of acidophilus directly into your vagina once a day, or use a rubber bulb syringe to insert one tablespoon of liquid culture. Another possibility would be tea tree oil, a nontoxic treatment very useful for fungal infections. You can find it in health food or herb stores. Mix 1 1/2 tablespoons of the oil in a cup of warm water and use it as a douche once a day. If you experience any irritation, however, discontinue its use.

Can Zinc Cure the Common Cold?

Q:
I've heard some talk about zinc lozenges as a cure for the common cold. Is there any validity to this claim? If it's true, where can I find the lozenges?

A:
Zinc gluconate lozenges do have a lot of enthusiasts, although in my experience, reports from users vary. Research on zinc has also delivered mixed results, but one recent study at the Cleveland Clinic found the mineral to cut the duration of a cold in half. No one, however, has found a cure for the common cold.

In the Cleveland study, 50 people with colds sucked on Cold-Eeze lozenges (13 milligrams each) every two hours. Their symptoms cleared up four days sooner than the coughing, runny noses, and sore throats of a comparable group that didn't use the lozenges. Michael Macknin, who designed the research, thinks the zinc ions traveled from the mouth to the nose, where they prevented the viruses that cause colds from settling into the respiratory pathways.

You should be aware that daily doses of zinc above 100 milligrams may depress immunity. And zinc can upset some people's stomachs, so make sure you've eaten before sucking on the lozenges. A lot of people don't like the taste of the lozenges, either.

I personally haven't experienced great benefits from zinc lozenges, but I think they are worth trying. You can buy them in health food stores or regular drugstores. Some say that the newer zinc acetate lozenges work better than standard forms.

Resources

Books by Andrew Weil, M.D.

Eight Weeks to Optimum Health: A Proven Program for Taking Full Advantage of Your Body's Natural Healing Power. New York: Alfred A. Knopf, 1997.

Spontaneous Healing: How to Discover and Enhance Your Body's Natural Ability to Maintain and Heal Itself. New York: Ballantine Books, 1996.

Natural Health, Natural Medicine: A Comprehensive Manual for Wellness and Self-Care. Rev. ed. Boston: Houghton Mifflin, 1995.

Health and Healing: Understanding Conventional and Alternative Medicine. Rev. ed. Boston: Houghton Mifflin, 1995.

From Chocolate to Morphine: Everything You Need to Know About Mind-Altering Drugs, with Winifred Rosen. Rev. ed. Boston: Houghton Mifflin, 1993.

The Natural Mind: An Investigation of Drugs and the Higher Consciousness. Rev. ed. Boston: Houghton Mifflin, 1986.

The Marriage of the Sun and Moon: A Quest for Unity in Consciousness. Boston: Houghton Mifflin, 1980.

Other Recommended Books

Barry, Diana. *Nips & Tucks: Everything You Must Know Before Having Cosmetic Surgery.* Los Angeles: General Publishing Group, 1996.

Becker, Robert O. *Cross Currents: The Perils of Electropollution, the Promise of Electromedicine.* Los Angeles: Jeremy Tarcher, 1990; dist. by St. Martin's Press.

Benson, Herbert. *The Relaxation Response.* New York: William Morrow, 1975.

Bruun, Ruth Dowling, and Bertel Bruun. *A Mind of Its Own. Tourette's Syndrome: A Story and a Guide.* New York: Oxford University Press, 1994.

Chang, Jolan. *The Tao of Love and Sex: The Ancient Chinese Way to Ecstasy.* New York: Viking Penguin, 1991.

Chang, Jolan. *The Tao of the Loving Couple.* New York: Dutton, 1995.

Chester, Laura. *Lupus Novice: Towards Self-Healing.* Barrytown, New York: Station Hill Press, 1987.

Fulford, Robert C., and Gene Stone. *Dr. Fulford's Touch of Life: The Healing Power of the Natural Life Force.* New York: Pocket Books, 1996.

Hallam, Richard. *Tinnitus: Dealing with the Ringing in Your Ears.* London: Thorsons, 1993.

Keville, Kathi, with Peter Korn. *Herbs for Health and Healing: The Illustrated Encyclopedia of Herbs.* Emmaus, Pennsylvania: Rodale Press, 1996.

Lerner, Michael. *Choice in Healing: Integrating the Best of Conventional and Alternative Approaches to Cancer.* Cambridge: MIT Press, 1994.

Northrup, Christiane, M.D. *Women's Bodies, Women's Wisdom: Creating Physical and Emotional Health and Healing.* New York: Bantam Books, 1995.

Reiter, Russel J., and Jo Robinson. *Melatonin: Your Body's Natural Wonder Drug.* New York: Bantam Books, 1995.

Sacks, Oliver. *The Man Who Mistook His Wife for a Hat.* New York: Summit Books, 1985.

Sahelian, Ray, M.D. *DHEA: A Practical Guide.* Garden City Park, New York: Avery Publishing Group, 1996.

Sarno, John, M.D. *Healing Back Pain: The Mind-Body Connection.* New York: Warner Books, 1991.

Schwartz, Cheryl. *Four Paws, Five Directions.* Berkeley: Celestial Arts, 1996.

Washnis, George J., and Richard Z. Hricak. *Discovery of Magnetic Health: A Health Care Alternative.* Rockville, Maryland: Nova Publishing, 1993.

Other Resources

American Association of Naturopathic Physicians
601 Valley Street, Suite 105
Seattle, WA 98109
206 298-0125

American Cancer Society
1599 Clifton Road
Atlanta, GA 30329
800 ACS-2345 (227-2345)

American Tinnitus Foundation
P.O. Box 5
Portland, OR 97207
503 248-9985

Biofeedback Certification Institute of America
10200 West 44th Avenue, Suite 304
Wheat Ridge, CO 80033
303 420-2902

Eclectic Institute
14385 Southeast Lusted Road
Sandy, OR 97055
503 668-4120 or 800 332-4372
Fax: 503 668-3227

EPA Safe Drinking Water Hotline
800 426-4791

Heintzman Farms
R.R. 2, Box 265
Onaka, SD 57466
605 447-5813

Home Access
800 HIV TEST (448-8378)

In Life Energy Systems
107 California Avenue
Mill Valley, CA 94941
415 389-1738

L&H Vitamins
37-10 Crescent Street
Long Island City, NY 11101
800 221-1152

National Abortion and Reproductive Rights Action League
1156 15th Street NW, Suite 700
Washington, DC 20005
202 973-3000

National Organization for SAD
P.O. Box 40133
Washington, DC 20016

National Radon Hotline
800 767-7236

National Sleep Foundation
1367 Connecticut Avenue NW, Suite 200
Washington, DC 20036
202 785-2300

New Day Films
201 652-6590

Planned Parenthood Federation of America
810 Seventh Avenue
New York, NY 10019
800 230-PLAN

The Population Council
One Dag Hammarskjöld Plaza
New York, NY 10017
212 339-0500
Fax: 212 755-6052

Rolf Institute
205 Canyon Boulevard
Boulder, CO 80302
303 449-5903 or 800 530-8875
Fax: 303 449-5978

Tourette Syndrome Association
42-40 Bell Boulevard
Bayside, NY 11361
718 224-2999

Vance's DariFree
800 275-1437

The Vitamin Shoppe
4700 Westside Avenue
North Bergen, NJ 07047
800 223-1216

Program in Integrative Medicine

At the University of Arizona Health Sciences Center, Tucson, Arizona. For more information, visit the Web site: http://www.ahsc.arizona.edu/integrative_medicine. Or write: Center for Integrative Medicine, P.O. Box 64089, Tucson, AZ 85718.

Newsletter

If you would like more information on my lectures and informational products, including my monthly newsletter, *Self Healing,* please write to: Andrew Weil, M.D., P.O. Box 457, Vail, AZ 85641.

On the Web

"Ask Dr. Weil" answers health questions daily on Time Warner's Pathfinder Network (www.drweil.com).

Index

About the Author

ANDREW WEIL, M.D., a graduate of Harvard College and Harvard Medical School, worked for the National Institute of Mental Health and for fifteen years was a research associate in ethnopharmacology at the Harvard Botanical Museum. As a fellow of the Institute of Current World Affairs, he traveled extensively throughout the world collecting information about medicinal plants and healing. He is the founder of the Center for Integrative Medicine in Tucson, Arizona, and director of the Program in Integrative Medicine at the University of Arizona.

About the Editor

STEVEN PETROW is the executive producer of the "Ask Dr. Weil" program. Mr. Petrow has held editorial positions with *Life* magazine, *Longevity* magazine, *Fitness*, and *The Wall Street Journal*. He has also been the editor in chief of *10 Percent* magazine and *AIDS Digest* and has published five books, including *The HIV Drug Book* and *When Someone You Know Has AIDS*.

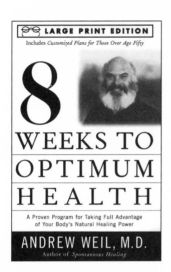

Look for these and other Random House Large Print books at your local bookstore

Angelou, Maya, *Even the Stars Look Lonesome*

Berendt, John, *Midnight in the Garden of Good and Evil*

Brinkley, David, *Everyone Is Entitled to My Opinion*

Carr, Caleb, *The Angel of Darkness*

Carter, Jimmy, *Living Faith*

Carter, Jimmy, *Sources of Strength*

Chopra, Deepak, *Ageless Body, Timeless Mind*

Chopra, Deepak, *The Path to Love*

Crichton, Michael, *Airframe*

Cronkite, Walter, *A Reporter's Life*

Daley, Rosie, *In the Kitchen with Rosie*

Flagg, Fannie, *Daisy Fay and the Miracle Man*

Flagg, Fannie, *Fried Green Tomatoes at the Whistle Stop Cafe*

Hepburn, Katharine, *Me*

Hiaasen, Carl, *Lucky You*

James, P. D., *A Certain Justice*

Koontz, Dean, *Sole Survivor*

Landers, Ann, *Wake Up and Smell the Coffee!*

le Carré, John, *The Tailor of Panama*

Lindbergh, Anne Morrow, *Gift from the Sea*

Mayle, Peter, *Chasing Cézanne*

Morrison, Toni, *Paradise*

Mother Teresa, *A Simple Path*

Patterson, Richard North, *Silent Witness*

Peck, M. Scott, M.D., *Denial of the Soul*

Phillips, Louis, editor, *The Random House Large Print Treasury of Best-Loved Poems*

Powell, Colin with Joseph E. Persico, *My American Journey*

Preston, Richard, *The Cobra Event*

Rampersad, Arnold, *Jackie Robinson*

Shaara, Jeff, *Gods and Generals*

Snead, Sam with Fran Pirozzolo, *The Game I Love*

Truman, Margaret, *Murder in the House*

Tyler, Anne, *Ladder of Years*

Updike, John, *Golf Dreams*

Weil, Andrew, M.D., *Eight Weeks to Optimum Health*